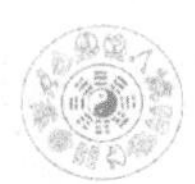

中华传统医学文化教育与普及丛书

中医名著

Masterpieces of Traditional Chinese Medicine

（汉英对照）

吕翠田 著
朱文晓 金 雪 主 译
许二平 中文主审
张加民 英文主审

东南大学出版社
SOUTHEAST UNIVERSITY PRESS
·南京·

内 容 提 要

《中医名著》对中国历史上具有重要影响的医学典籍的主要内容、学术思想做了整理，涉及内、外、伤、妇、小儿等各科，重点介绍了这些典籍的学术特点以及在中医史上的突出地位和重要贡献，以帮助读者了解中医不同流派、不同时期的学术特点，进一步加深对中医发展、流变的认识，并从此角度更加深刻地理解中医，从而为进一步深入学习研究奠定基础。

本书适用于从事中医学习、研究及对中医或中国传统文化有兴趣的人员，也可作为汉语国际教育、来华外国留学生及中国传统文化推广的教材使用。

图书在版编目(CIP)数据

中医名著：汉英对照／吕翠田著；朱文晓，金雪主译. —南京：东南大学出版社，2018.6

ISBN 978-7-5641-7708-9

Ⅰ.①中… Ⅱ.①吕… ②朱… ③金… Ⅲ.①医论-汇编-中国-汉、英 Ⅳ.①R249.1

中国版本图书馆 CIP 数据核字(2018)第 069261 号

中医名著(汉英对照)

著 者	吕翠田	责任编辑	刘 坚
主 译	朱文晓 金 雪		
电 话	(025)83793329 QQ:635353748	电子邮件	liu-jian@seu.edu.cn
出版发行	东南大学出版社	出 版 人	江建中
地 址	南京市四牌楼 2 号(210096)	邮 编	210096
销售电话	(025)83794561/83794174/83794121/83795801/83792174/83795802/57711295(传真)		
网 址	http://www.seupress.com	电子邮件	press@seupress.com
经 销	全国各地新华书店	印 刷	虎彩印艺股份有限公司
开 本	787mm×1092mm 1/16	印 张	10.5 字 数 305 千字
版 次	2018 年 6 月第 1 版	印 次	2018 年 6 月第 1 次印刷
书 号	ISBN 978-7-5641-7708-9		
定 价	40.00 元		

总序

人类在漫长的发展进程中创造了丰富多彩的文明，中华文明是世界文明多样性、多元化的重要组成部分，对世界文明进步产生了积极影响。中医药是中华优秀传统文化的典型代表，强调道法自然、天人合一、阴阳平衡、调和致中，体现了中华文化的内核。中医药还提倡"辨证论治"，"仁心仁术"，更丰富了中华文化内涵，为中华民族认识和改造世界提供了有益启迪。

中医药的文化内涵和学术价值也越来越为世人接纳和认可。目前已有130个中医药类项目列入国家级非物质文化遗产代表性项目名录，"中医针灸"列入联合国教科文组织人类非物质文化遗产代表作名录，《黄帝内经》和《本草纲目》入选世界记忆名录。屠呦呦因发现"青蒿素——一种用于治疗疟疾的药物"，荣获2011年美国拉斯克临床医学奖和2015年诺贝尔生理学或医学奖。因将传统中药的砷剂与西药结合而显著提高急性早幼粒细胞白血病的疗效，王振义、陈竺获得第七届圣捷尔吉癌症研究创新成就奖。

在"一带一路"背景下的今天，中医药文化的国际发展尤其引人瞩目。然而这套丛书的目的不在于把中医药文化拿出去给世人看，乃是邀请世人走进中医药的世界，一起来领略天覆地载、万物悉备中的春生夏长、秋收冬藏、君臣佐使、浮沉升降，体味在这个古老的东方国度里某些生活态度和思维方式何以形成，人们与自然如何彼此相应。

这套丛书共分四册：《中医理论》将带你进入中医药独特的思维方式和理论体系中。在这里，你将认识一对对概念，如天与地、上与下、内与外、昼与夜、明与暗、寒与热、虚与实、散与聚，既相互对立，又在此消彼长中获得动态的平衡。你也将领略金木水火土之间的运动变化、相生相克，以及五行如何从五种具体物质中抽象出来，上升为哲学的理性概念。在这里，心为君主，肺为相傅，肝为将军，脾胃为仓廪之官；在这里，你会看到有形的五脏和无形的经络；你将看到中医如何"视其外应，测知其内"，并学会如何"顺时摄养"，保持机体内外环境的协调统一。

《中医名言》是历代名家名言的集锦，许多隽永的句子今天依然闪烁着智慧的光芒。这里有丰富的医学人文思想："医，仁术也。仁人君子，必笃于情。"无恒德者，不可以作医。也有对生命的尊重："人命至重，有贵千金，一方济之，德逾于此。"许多名言简洁而练达，言有尽而意无穷，有种不可言说的美感：坚者削之、客者除之、劳者温之、结者散之、留者攻之、燥者濡之、散者收之、损者温之、逸者行之、惊者平之、微者逆之、甚者从之……

《中医名家》对历代名医进行了介绍，包括生平简介、医学贡献、学术思想以及趣闻轶事等等，使读者从更加直观具体的角度来了解中医学的思想，而且每个医家各有所长，如清朝叶桂所言"内伤必取法乎东垣"（《叶氏医案存真》）。你在这里会深入了解很多名医，如孙思邈、华佗、扁鹊、张仲景、王叔和、葛洪等，也会结识一些普通人不太熟悉但是有过突出贡献的医生：薛己、缪希雍、喻昌等。有些是宫廷御医，有些却游走于民间市井街巷，有些出身名门，有些家境贫寒，他们以高尚的医德和精湛的医术使他们的影响超越了时代和国界。

《中医名著》对有代表性的历代中医典籍的主要内容、学术思想做了整理。其中，《黄帝内经》是中医理论体系的奠基之作，被奉为"医家之宗"；《伤寒杂病论》是我国医学在临床方面获得迅速发展的一个重要标志。你还将看到我国第一部医学百科全书——《千金方》，中医第一部临床急救手册——《肘后备急方》，最早的针灸学专著——《针灸甲乙经》，我国现存最早的药物学专著——《神农本草经》，中医关于药物炮制的第一部专书——《雷公炮炙论》，以及几百年来令医学界争论不休的《医林改错》……

没有任何一门学科的语言像中医语言一样有如此丰富的修辞：逆水行舟、闭门留寇、滋水涵木、提壶揭盖、釜底抽薪；治上焦如羽，非轻不举；治下焦如权，非重不沉。

也没有哪门学科的术语具备如此和谐的音节和对仗的词语：盛者责之，虚者责之；郁火宜发，实火宜泻；发表不远热，攻里不远寒；攻不可以收缓功，补不可以求速效。

中医哲学的深邃思想也体现在字里行间，在望闻问切、理法方药中，往往有更多哲理的意蕴：天地之理，有开必有合；用药之机，有补必有泻；见病医病，医家大忌；急则治其标，缓则治其本。

在这个世界里，万物是彼此关联的：寒极生热，热极生寒；乙癸同源，肝肾同治；有诸内者，必形诸外。

在这个世界中，人与天地自然的关系是和谐的，人们日出而作，日落而息。阴阳自和者，必自愈。

在这个世界里，医生不只是医生，可以是统帅千军的将领，因为"用药如用兵"。善用兵者，必先屯粮；善治邪者，必先养正。其高者，因而越之；其下者，引而竭之；其在皮者，汗而发之；其慓悍者，按而收之；其实者，散而泻之。用补之法，贵乎先轻后重，务在成功；用攻之法，必须先缓后峻，及病则已。

在这个世界里，并非有病的人才需要医生，也并非能治病的人就是最好的医生，因为圣人"不治已病治未病，不治已乱治未乱"。病也远不仅仅出于风、寒、暑、湿、燥、火，还有喜、怒、忧、思、悲、恐、惊。

虽然中医是崇尚经典的：医之为书，非《素问》无以立论，非《本草》无以主方。然而这套丛书的目的绝不在于怀旧或尚古，而在于启发我们今天的生活，因为"善言天者，必有验于人；善言古者，必有合于今；善言人者，必有厌于己。"

"未医彼病，先医我心。"今天的社会充满了浮躁和喧哗，亲爱的读者，在走近这套丛书的时候，请先预备一颗安静的心。有医术，更要有医道。术可暂行一时，道则永远流传。这套丛书未必要培养高明的医者，但其中蕴含的生命哲理或能伴你一生。

李照国

于2017年8月

Preface

Humanity has created a colorful civilization in the long course of development, and the civilization of China is an important component of the diverse world civilization, producing a positive impact on the progress of human civilization. TCM is the epitome of traditional Chinese culture. Applying such principles as "man should observe the law of nature and seek for the unity of the heaven and humanity", "yin and yang should be balanced to obtain the golden mean". TCM embodies the core value of Chinese civilization. TCM also advocates "syndrome differentiation and treatment", and "mastership of medicine lying in proficient medical skills and lofty medical ethics", which enriches Chinese culture and provides an enlightened base for Chinese to study and transform the world.

TCM's cultural connotation and academic value are increasingly gaining acceptance around the world. Up till now, 130 TCM elements have been incorporated into the Representative List of National Intangible Cultural Heritage, with TCM acupuncture and moxibustion been included in the Representative List of the Intangible Cultural Heritage of Humanity by UNESCO, and *Huangdi's Internal Classic* and *Compendium of Materia Medica* are listed in the Memory of the World Register. Tu Youyou won the 2011 Lasker Award in clinical medicine and the 2015 Nobel Prize in Physiology or Medicine for discovering qinghaosu (artemisinin) to cure malaria. Wang Zhenyi and Chen Zhu were awarded the Seventh Annual Szent-Gyorgyi Prize for Progress in Cancer Research for combining the Western medicine ATRA and the TCM compound arsenic trioxide to treat acute promyelocytic leukemia (APL).

Under the background of "One Belt One Road Initiative", the global development of TCM has been put under the spotlight. Yet the motivation of the series is not to show TCM to the world, but to bring people to get into the world of TCM, to explore the realm with the covering of the heavens in the upper and the support of the earth in the lower, with the generating spring, growing summer, harvesting autumn and storing winter; and to comprehend the monarch, minister, assistant and guide (metaphors of medicines based on their functions) and the floating, sinking, ascending and descending of Chinese herbs; to have a taste of the way that styles of life and ways of thinking are formed, and how they adjust themselves to achieve the harmony with the environment in this ancient oriental kingdom.

The series include four books: *Basic Theory of TCM* will bring you into a unique way of thinking and the system of TCM theory. Here you will get to know a set of opposite concepts, such as the heaven and the earth, up and down, inside and outside, day and night, light and dark, cold and heat, deficiency and excess, the scattered and the gathered, yet are in dynamic balance through constant waxing and waning. You will also get to know the movement and change, promotion and restriction of wood, fire, earth, metal and water and see how the five elements are abstracted from the five materials and sublimated into philosophical rational concept. Here the heart is like a monarch, the lung is an assistant, the liver is a general, and the spleen and stomach are barn officials; here you will see the tangible five zang-organs and feel the intangible meridian system. You will know how the TCM doctors know the inside by observing the outside and how to regulate the spirit according to the changes of the four seasons to harmonize the internal and external environments of the body.

TCM Mottos is a collection of the famous sayings in TCM history, many of which are still glittering with the light of wisdom. Here you will read rich thoughts of medical humanities, "Medicine is a kind of compassionate skill. Benevolent gentlemen should be affectionate. Without solid morality, a person cannot become a doctor." It also shows the respect for human lives, "Human life is topmost and valuable, while a treatable formula is much more valuable." With their simplicity and expressiveness, the sayings here are inexpressibly beautiful with few words but infinite meanings: Diseases caused by hardness of qi should be treated with reducing therapy; invasion of evil should be treated with eliminating therapy. Overstrain should be treated with warming therapy; stagnation should be treated with dispersing therapy. Retention disease should be treated with attacking therapy. Dryness disease should be treated with moistening therapy. Flaccidity disease should be treated with astringing therapy. Impairment disease should be treated with warming therapy. Stagnancy disease should be treated with dredging therapy. Fright should be treated with calming therapy. Mild disease should be treated with contrary therapy; severe disease should be treated with conforming therapy...

Masters of TCM is an introduction of the famous doctors in Chinese history, including their lives, medical contribution, academic thoughts and anecdotes. You will learn about the TCM thinking from a more concrete and personal perspective. Each doctor has his own specialty, just as Ye Gui says, "To find treatment methods of internal diseases, all doctors refer to Li Dongyuan." (*Yeshi Yi'an Cunzhen*, written by Ye Gui of the Qing Dynasty) Here you will learn about some not so familiar names like Xue Ji, Miao Xiyong, Yu Chang, as well as some famous ones like Sun Simiao, Hua Tuo, Bian Que, Zhang Zhongjing, Wang Shuhe, and Ge Hong. Some of them were court physicians, yet others worked in villages and towns; some were born to the purple, yet some were of very humble-birth, whose influence all go beyond time and borders owing to their noble morality and outstanding medical skills.

Masterpieces of TCM introduces the content and academic value of some important TCM works in the history of Chinese medicine. *Huangdi's Internal Classic* lays the foundation of TCM theoretical system, thus it is called "the source of medical thoughts". *Treatise on Cold Damage and Miscellaneous Diseases* is a symbol of China's rapid development in clinical medicine. You will also read about the first medical encyclopedia in China——*Thousand Golden Prescriptions*, the first clinical first-aid manual of traditional Chinese medicine—*Handbook of Prescriptions for Emergency*, the earliest extant book on acupuncture and moxibustion *A-B Classic of Acupuncture and Moxibustion*, the earliest classic on materia medica extant in China——*Shennong's Classic of*

Materia Medica, the first monograph on processing of drugs——*Master Lei's Discourse on Medicine Processing*, and the book with endless arguments for hundreds of years in the medical world——*Correction on Errors in Medical Works*...

No other discipline has the language like TCM with so rich rhetorical expressions: sailing against the current, closing the door to keep the intruders, replenishing water to nourish wood, raising the kettle and opening the lid, taking away the firewood from under the cauldron; the disease of the upper energizer should be treated by drugs with light, clear, ascending and float natures, while the disease of the lower energizer should be treated by heavy, suppressing, greasy, nourishing and subduing drugs, which can affect the lower part of the body.

No other discipline has the terms with such melody in sound and symmetry in words: Diseases, be there symptoms excessive or deficient, should be explored from the root cause. Stagnant fire should be dispersed; excessive fire should be treated by clearing heat and reducing fire. When relieving pathogenic factors from the exterior, the use of drugs hot in nature should not be avoided; when attacking the interior, the use of drugs cold in nature should not be avoided. Attacking the pathogen should not be too slow, while nourishing should not be too rapid and effective.

The profound philosophical wisdom is often embodied in the simple TCM expressions. In the four examinations, the theories, treatments, formulas and drugs, you can draw deeper lessons: change in the world including opening and closing process; the mechanism of prescription including tonifying and purifying. Doctors should abstain from treating the exterior symptoms of the disease, but relieving the secondary in an urgent case and removing the primary in a chronic case.

In this world, everything is closely related with each other: Extreme cold generates heat and extreme heat produces cold. Yi (the second heavenly stem) and Gui (the tenth heavenly stem) have the same origin, which means that the liver and the kidney should be treated together. Every change inside the body is certainly manifested outside correspondingly.

In this world, human beings have a harmonious relationship with the nature: People get up to work when the sun rises and have rest when the sun sets. If yin and yang become harmonized by themselves, the disease will be cured.

In this world, doctors are more than doctors, but also commanders of the army since "treatment and prescription are similar to the command of military forces in the war". A general good at leading army will certainly store enough provisions to conserve energy and build up strength. A skillful doctor will certainly support and protect the vital qi when he is treating the disease and eliminating the pathogens. If the pathogenic factors have accumulated in the upper, vomiting therapy should be used. If the pathogenic factors have accumulated in the lower, dredging therapy should be used. If the pathogenic factors are in the skin, sweating therapy can be used. If the pathogenic conditions are acute, measures should be taken to control them. For excess or sthenia syndrome, dispersing therapy and purging therapy can be used. The treatment of invigoration should be light first and heavy then. The purgative method should be moderate first and fierce then.

In this world, not only the patients need doctors, and the best doctor is not the one who can treat diseases, since sages usually pay less attention to the treatment of a disease, but more to the prevention of it. They deal with problems before they appear, instead of dealing with them after they have appeared. Diseases are not only caused by wind, cold, heat, dampness, dryness and fire, but also joy, anger, worry, thinking, sorrow, fear and fright.

Although TCM greatly honors classic works: medical books are rooted in theories of *Su Wen* and based on formulas of *Compendium of Material Medica*, the purpose of the series is far from nostalgia or archaism, because "Those who are good at explaining the heavens must be able to prove it with human affairs, those who are good at discussing history must be able to relate it to the present situation and those who are good at talking about others must be able to delineate themselves."

Before curing diseases, doctors should keep their own mind correct first. Anyone who is going to open the series should bear a peaceful mind although today's society is filled with restlessness and noise. Medical doctrines always go before medical skills. Medical skills are used only for a time, while medical doctrines last through ages. This series of books will not necessarily equip you to be a qualified doctor, but the philosophy of life in them may benefit you for the rest of your life.

Li Zhaoguo

August, 8,2017

目录
CONTENTS

1 黄帝内经(Huangdi Neijing)

Huangdi's Internal Classic

一 书籍简介

《黄帝内经》(《内经》)是我国现存医学文献中最早、比较全面系统阐述中医学理论体系的古典医学巨著,奠定了中医学的理论基础,建立了中医学的理论体系。该书大约成书于西汉末期,具体年代不详,目前根据历史资料考证,推测该书的成书时间为公元前一世纪内。全书包括《素问》和《灵枢》两部分,每部分9卷,每卷有9篇,共计162篇。

该书的作者被认为非黄帝所作,但是为何冠之以“黄帝”二字?原来在中国的古代传说中,“黄帝”是一个远古时期的君王,也是中国中原地区部落百姓的共同祖先;另有说法认为黄帝不是一个人,而是一个伟大的部落氏族——黄帝族,在中国的中部地区定居生活,也被称为“华族”,是中华民族的始祖,也是“汉族”的祖先。人们一般为突出祖先传承的延续,常将一切文化追溯至黄帝,在本书成书的时期,当时的学者为了凸显学有根本,将著作托名“黄帝”所著,以示重要。

1 A brief introduction to the book

Huangdi's Internal Classic (*Huangdi Neijing*) is the earliest extant medical classic in China, which gives a comprehensive and systematic exposition of the theoretical system of Traditional Chinese Medicine (TCM). It lays the theoretical foundation and establishes the theoretical system of TCM. It appeared approximately in the late Western Han Dynasty, but the exact time is uncertain. According to historical records, it was speculated that the book was compiled before the 1st century B. C. The book consists of two parts: *Plain Questions* and *Miraculous Pivot*. Each part comprises nine volumes and each volume contains nine chapters, totaling up to 162 chapters.

It is believed that the book was not written by Huangdi, then why was it named after Huangdi? According to the ancient Chinese legends, Huangdi was an emperor in antiquity as well as the common ancestor of tribes in the central plains of China. Another saying was that Huangdi was not a specific person, but a great clan—Huangdi Clan, also called Hua Zu, the ancestor of Chinese nation and the Han nationality, who inhabited in central China. In order to emphasize the continuity of ancestral inheritance, people often traced all the culture back to Huangdi. That the book was entitled in this way during its compilation could highlight the solid foundation of the study and reflect its value and authority.

这种做法也是一种当时流行的做法,不少古代的著作都托名"黄帝",如《黄帝说》、《黄帝阴阳》等。《内经》的"经"是经典的意思,也被解释为常道、规范的意思,大凡在古代中医文献中,被称为"经"的著作都可以视作医学的规范,让从医的人员所学习和遵循的。"内"是与"外"相对而言的,古代文献书名中的内或者外,类似现在书籍的上下篇或者上下部。

This practice was quite common at that time. Many other classics also employed this practice, such as *The Legends of Huangdi* (*Huangdi Shuo*) *Huangdi's Yin and Yang* (*Huangdi Yinyang*), etc. The Chinese character "Jing" in *Huangdi's Internal Classic* refers to classics or the normal laws and principles. Among the ancient TCM literature, classics with the name of "Jing" are taken as the medical norms for medical workers to learn and follow. Nei (inside) is contrary to Wai (outside). "Nei" or "Wai" in the names of ancient classics is similar to different chapters or volumes in present books.

二 主要内容

《黄帝内经》一书中的内容非常丰富,除了医学知识以外,还包括总结了秦汉以前天文、历法、气象、地理、心理、生物等众多学科的内容,可以说汲取和融会了古代哲学、自然科学的成就,从宏观角度论述了天地人之间的相互联系,讨论和分析了医学科学最基本的课题——生命规律,并创建了相应的理论体系和防治疾病的原则和技术。目前认为《黄帝内经》中的医学理论内容可分为养生、阴阳五行、藏象、气血精神、经络、病因病机、病症、诊法、论治和运气十类。

2 The main content

Huangdi's Internal Classic is rich in its content. Apart from medical knowledge, it also summarizes many other subjects in ancient times, such as astronomy, calendar, meteorology, geography, psychology and biology, etc. As a collection and combination of the ancient achievements in philosophy and natural science, it analyzes the interrelation of heaven, earth and people from the macroscopic view, discusses the most basic medical issue—the law of life and establishes the corresponding theoretical system and the principles and technology of disease prevention and treatment. At present, it is considered that the medical theory in the book can fall into ten categories: health-cultivation, yin, yang and five elements, visceral manifestations, meridians and collaterals, qi, blood, essence and spirit, etiology and pathogenesis, syndrome, diagnosis, treatment and qi circulation.

① 养生部分主要突出"不治已病治未病"的预防思想,提出人们可以通过顺应自然规律变化,情志恬静淡泊,不为欲望所困,在饮食上

① The part of health cultivation mainly emphasizes "less attention to the treatment of a disease, but more to the prevention of it". Accordingly, people should be in conformity with the regular change of the nature, cultivating a healthy lifestyle to keep the mind peaceful and calm,

有规律，不可偏食，各种食物要食用合理得当，起居劳作要适度，不可过度劳累，并积极参加导引等活动而促进身体健康，以达延年益寿目的。

restraining the desire, keeping regular and balanced diet and avoiding overwork. Furthermore, people should take some exercises actively such as *Daoyin*(a kind of exercise used to cultivate health and cure disease through moving the limbs and regulating breath) to keep fit and prolong life.

② 阴阳五行部分主要从医学角度阐释了古代哲学思想中的阴阳和五行观点，认为阴阳观是世界宇宙变化运动发展的内在基本规律，万事万物都具有阴阳矛盾和受阴阳变化的影响，人的生命活动也离不开阴阳的相互制约和相互促进，阴阳平衡是人体健康的状态，而阴阳失调则是疾病发生、发展和变化的基本机制。同时认为五行观也是世界宇宙变化运动发展的内在基本规律，整个世界都归属于五行生化的系统，人体内的脏器、官窍、肢体、情志等也都分别归属于五行的功能系统，从而形成了对人体整体功能系统的认识。

② The part of yin, yang and five elements mainly expounds the concepts of yin, yang and five elements in the ancient philosophical thoughts from the medical viewpoint. It believes that yin-yang concept is the internal basic law of the universal change, movement and development. All things in the world embody the yin-yang contradiction and are influenced by the change of yin and yang. Life activities cannot be separated from the mutual restriction and promotion of yin and yang. The balance of yin and yang reflects the healthy status of the human body, while the imbalance of yin and yang functions as the basic mechanism of the occurrence, development and change of diseases. Moreover, the concept of five elements is also an internal basic law of the universal change, movement and development. The whole world can be categorized into the system of generation and transformation of five elements. Viscera, orifices, limbs and emotions are all attributed to the functional system of five elements, thus forming the recognition of the holistic functional system of the human body.

③ 藏象部分主要研究人体的内在脏器功能和所显现出的生理功能之间的联系，以心肝脾肺肾五脏为中心，将其他脏器、四肢、官窍等分属五大功能系统，并通过经络的沟通，气血的贯通流注而形成整体。藏象学说是《内经》理论体系的核心，也是临床中医诊

③ The part of visceral manifestation mainly covers the connection between internal human organs and their physiological functions. Centered on five zang-organs (heart, liver, spleen, lung and kidney), other organs, four limbs and orifices are classified into five functional systems and then integrate into a whole through the connection of meridians and collaterals and flow of qi and blood. The visceral manifestation theory is the core of the theoretical system of *Internal Classic* and also the important theoretical

治疾病的重要理论基础。

basis of clinical diagnosis and treatment of diseases.

④ 气血精神部分论述了气血是维持人体生命活动的最基本物质。精是生命的本源，是来自于父母的生命物质和后天生命体内的精微生命物质融合成的人体精华，也是维持人体生命活动的基本物质。神包括人的精神活动如不同的情绪和不同的意识状态以及调控生命活动的高级系统。

④ The part of qi, blood, essence and spirit holds that qi and blood are the most basic substance of maintaining human life activities. Essence is the origin of life, coming from body essence integrated by the parents' life substance and acquired subtle living matters in the body, which is also a basic substance of maintaining human life activities. The spirit includes human spiritual activities, such as different emotions and ideologies, as well as the advanced system that regulates the life activities.

⑤ 经络部分论述了分布在人体内的运行气血、沟通内外上下、联络脏腑组织器官的系统，这是人体内所存在的重要生理功能系统，为针灸技术的推行奠定了理论基础，具有重要的理论地位。

⑤ The part of meridians and collaterals talks about the internal system that helps to promote the circulation of qi and blood, communicate the interior and exterior, the upper and lower parts and combine tissues and organs. Being an important physiological functional system within the human body, it lays a theoretical foundation for the promotion of needling techniques and holds an important position in theory.

⑥ 病因病机部分主要阐释了疾病的病因以及疾病发生、发展和转归的规律，认为导致疾病发生的重要致病因素包括外在因素如气候反常变化和内在因素如个人的情志刺激变化等。对于发病提出了“正气存内，邪不可干”的重要观点，即强调人体的正气在预防发病中的重要作用。对于疾病的发展变化提出以邪正盛衰、阴阳失调等来解释疾病的基本机理。

⑥ The part of etiology and pathogenesis mainly illustrates the cause of diseases and the law of occurrence, development and transformation of diseases. It holds that significant pathogenic factors include external factors, such as the abnormal change of climate and the internal factors, such as the stimulation and change of personal emotions. As for the attack of diseases, this part puts forward an important view that "invasion of pathogenic factors will be avoided if there is sufficient vital qi (healthy qi) inside the body", which emphasizes the importance of vital qi in the prevention of diseases. As for the development and change of diseases, the basic mechanism of diseases can be explained by some corresponding syndromes, such as the excess and deficiency of vital qi and pathogenic qi, the imbalance of yin and yang, etc.

⑦ 在病症部分,《内经》记载了多达三百多个疾病种类,如咳嗽、热病、肿胀等,并有不少以病症为篇名的专论,如《咳论》、《痹论》等。

⑦ As for the syndromes, more than three hundred diseases are recorded in *Huangdi's Internal Classic*, such as cough, febrile diseases and swelling, etc. There are also many other monographs designated with syndromes, such as the *Discussion on Cough* and *Discussion on Impediment*.

⑧ 诊法方面论述了中医的望、闻、问、切四种诊断方法,尤其对于望诊中的望色和切脉有详细的描述,如通过观察面部色泽的变化来推断疾病及其预后情况;并详细阐述了切脉的方法、脉象所主的疾病和诊脉的注意事项等内容,为后世中医脉诊的研究提供了基础。

⑧ Four diagnostic methods are discussed in this book, namely *wang* (observing), *wen* (listening), *wen* (inquiring) and *qie* (pulse-taking). Among them, *wang* (observing) and *qie* (pulse-taking) are described in detail, such as observing the change of facial complexion to speculate diseases and the prognosis of diseases. It also expounds the pulse-taking methods, cautions and pulse-related diseases, providing a basis for the later study of TCM pulse-taking examination.

⑨ 论治方面主要讲述了对疾病的治疗方法和治疗原则。《内经》所记载的治疗方法很多,如砭石、针刺、药物、熏洗、按摩、饮食疗法等。在治疗原则方面指出治疗的根本目的是调和阴阳平衡,注重人体的整体联系,强调"治病必求其本"的原则,分清疾病的轻重缓急,并结合季节气候、地区环境以及个体差异而制定适宜的治疗方案。

⑨ The part of disease treatment mainly describes the treatment methods and principles. There are many treatments recorded in *Internal Classic*, such as stone needling, acupuncture, medication, fumigation-washing therapy, massage and dietary treatment, etc. With regard to treatment principles, the book points out that the basic purpose of treatment is to regulate yin-yang balance, to focus on the overall connection of human body, emphasizing that "the treatment of disease must follow the origin". Therefore, therapeutic plans should be decided based on the consideration of the states of disease, seasons and climate, regional environment as well as individual differences.

⑩ 运气主要论述了古代的运气学说,即专门研究自然天象、气象的变化规律和对人类疾病发生流行的影响关系。运气学说作为古代的医学气象学,是《内经》理论体系的组成部分之一,对今天研究医学与气象学有一定参考价值。

⑩ The part of qi circulation mainly discusses the ancient *Yunqi* (Motion of Qi) theory, a specialized study of the influence of the astronomical phenomena and changing weather on human diseases. As an ancient medical meteorology, *Yunqi* theory is a part of the theoretical system of *Internal Classic*, which is still of certain value to the modern study of medicine and meteorology.

三 学术价值

（1）《黄帝内经》是中医理论体系的奠基之作

在《内经》问世以前，医学处于零星的不成系统的医学经验积累阶段，《内经》一书的形成，将医疗经验和当时先进的哲学思想融合，并升华为系统的理论体系，为中医学的发展提供了理论依据和指导方法，为历代医学家提供了医学理论原理。

两千多年来中医学的持续发展，正是与历代医学家在《内经》理论基础之上将《内经》理论实践、运用和探索、创新密不可分，因此《内经》被人们奉为"医家之宗"。《内经》之后，中医学术虽然代有发展，流派纷呈，医学著作汗牛充栋，然而追溯这些学说、流派和著作的渊源，无一不是来自《内经》。

（2）确立了"天—地—人"的医学模式

《内经》认为人是自然界的产物，人的生命现象也是自然现象的一部分，因此人的生命现象、活动规律与自然是一个不可分割的整体，都遵循着同一个自然规律。《内经》中要求作为医生，应该"上知天文，下知地理，中知人事"，"天文"、"地理"均指自然环境种种影响因素，"人事"泛指社会人际等事情，大到国家社会、

3 Academic value

(1) Laying the foundation of TCM theoretical system

Before the publication of *Internal Classic*, medical science was in an accumulating stage of sporadic, unsystematic experience. By combining medical experience with the advanced philosophical thoughts at that time, the book sublimates the experience to an organized theoretical system, offering the theoretical reference and instructions for TCM development and the principles of medical theories for generations of medical scientists.

The continual development of TCM over 2000 years closely owes to the practice, application, exploration and innovation of theories in *Internal Classic* on its theoretical basis, thus it is called "the source of medical thoughts". After the publication of *Internal Classic*, TCM has developed into many schools of theories, with numerous medical works produced. If we trace the origin, however, it can be found that all the theories, schools and works are from *Internal Classic*.

(2) Establishing the medical model of "heaven-earth-people"

According to *Internal Classic*, human beings are products of the nature. Human life is also a part of the natural phenomenon, thus human life and activities are inseparably combined with the nature, following the same natural law. *Internal Classic* demands that a doctor should have a good command of astronomy, geography and human activities. The astronomy and geography both mean the influential factors of the natural environment, while human activities generally refer to the social and interpersonal events, ranging from the big things related to the country, society, politics, economy, culture and folk custom to

政治经济文化、民风习俗等，小到个人的经济地位、家境遭遇和个人经历等，这些都与人体的心身健康有着密切关系。

这种医学模式与近代医学界所提出的“社会—心理—生物”医学模式的基本观点是相通的，即都不把人作为一个独立体，而是看作自然环境、社会环境中的一员。这种医学模式对于中医学的发展和治疗疾病的疗效有着深远的指导意义。

small events such as personal economic status, family environment and personal experience, etc. All these things are closely linked to the physical and mental health of the human body.

This medical model coincides with the bio-psycho-social model advocated by modern medical science, which views person as a member of the natural and social environment instead of an independent individual. It has profound guiding significance to the development of TCM and its curative effects.

(3) 对世界医学具有一定的影响

《内经》不仅是一部被国内医家所高度重视的经典医籍，而且对世界医学的发展亦有其不可忽略的影响。例如日本、朝鲜等国，都曾把《内经》列为医学生必读的课本。《素问》和《灵枢》的部分内容，也相继被翻译成日、英、德、法等国文字以供学习和研究。国外一些针灸学术组织，还把《内经》作为针灸医生的必读参考书。英国科学家李约瑟博士曾经这样评价说：“(《内经》)在综合《内经》成书时的中医状态，随着两千年土生土长的临床以后，仍然注定保持不变，相反有巨大的发展，有许多精心杰作和派生的学派。如果我们在想到中医有过任何献礼，作为一部经典著作应该受之不愧。”

(3) Producing certain impact on the world medicine

Internal Classic is not only a medical classic highly stressed by Chinese medical scientists, but also has a great influence on the development of the world medicine. For example, in Japan and Korea, *Internal Classic* has been listed as a compulsory textbook of the medical students. Partial contents in *Plain Questions* and *Miraculous Pivot* have also been successively translated into Japanese, English, German and French for study and research. Besides, some foreign academic organizations in acupuncture and moxibustion also took *Internal Classic* as the required reference book for acupuncture and moxibustion doctors. British scientist Dr. Joseph Needham (also called Li Yuese) once remarked, “It is hard to imagine that the comprehensive condition of TCM would still remain the same after 2000 years of indigenous clinical practice. On the contrary, it made huge development during which many schools and masterpieces came into being. If we could think about any contribution of TCM, *Huangdi's Internal Classic* undoubtedly deserves to be the one.”

2 难经(Nan Jing)

Classic of Difficult Issues

一 书籍简介

《难经》又名《黄帝八十一难经》,是《黄帝内经》以后的又一重要医籍。全书以阐明《内经》的要旨为主,用问答的体裁,共编辑为八十一难。对于《难经》的作者和成书年代素来有不同说法。据文献记载,最早提到《难经》书名的是东汉张仲景的《伤寒杂病论自序》,张仲景提到参考《八十一难》一书,但未写明该书的作者;至唐代才有了"《难经》的作者是战国时代的秦越人(扁鹊)"的说法,但多数人也不同意这种说法,因此作者不详。现在一般认为《难经》是东汉时的著作,成书年代在《内经》之后。《难经》书名之"难"字是何含义?一般有两种解释:一是问难,即指书中以问答为形式来阐述《内经》的深奥道理,有提出,质问之义;二是难易,即指本书的内容医理深远,非简单容易之义。

1 A brief introduction to the book

Classic of Difficult Issues (*Nan Jing*), also known as *Huangdi's Canon of Eighty-One Difficult Issues*, is an important medical classic after the appearance of *Huangdi's Internal Classic*. The book mainly clarifies the quintessence of *Internal Classic* in a question-and-answer format, in total 81 difficult issues. The opinions about the book's author and date of composition vary all the time. According to documentary records, the book was earliest mentioned in *Preface of Treatise on Cold Damage and Miscellaneous Diseases* (*Shanghan Zabing Lun Zixu*), which was written by Zhang Zhongjing in the Eastern Han Dynasty. In the preface, he mentioned that he referred to *Eighty-One Difficult Issues* (*Bashiyi Nan*), but made no mention of the book's author. It was not clear until the Tang Dynasty that there was a saying the author of *Classic of Difficult Issues* was Qin Yueren (Bian Que), a famous doctor in the Period of Warring States (475—221 B. C.). However, most people disagreed with it and the author still remained unknown. Now it is generally considered that the book was compiled in the Eastern Han Dynasty (25—220 A. D.) after *Internal Classic*. What is the meaning of "*Nan*" in the name of *Nan Jing*? Generally there are two kinds of explanations. One is query, which emphasizes the book elaborates on the enigmatic thought of *Internal Classic* in a question-and-answer form. The other one refers to difficulty, which means that the book is not easily understood since the content is too insightful.

二 主要内容

《难经》一书的内容是在《内经》基础上,提出了八十一个问题并进行重点讨论,内容涉及生理、病理、诊断和治疗等各个方面。其中"一至二十二难"为脉学的讨论,"二十三至二十九难"为经络的讨论,"三十至四十七难"为脏腑的讨论,"四十八至六十一难"为疾病的讨论,"六十二至六十八难"为腧穴的讨论,"六十九至八十一难"为针法的讨论。

2 The main content

On the basis of *Internal Classic*, *Classic of Difficult Issues* discusses eighty-one questions, which mainly includes different aspects about Chinese medicine, such as physiology, pathology, diagnosis and treatment of diseases. In this book, questions 1—22, 23—29 and 30—47 respectively deal with sphygmology, meridians and collaterals, and zang-fu organs; questions 48—61, 62—68 and 69—81 respectively explore diseases, acupoints, and acupuncture therapy.

(1) 关于脉学内容的阐述

和《内经》相比较,有关脉学的内容在《难经》中占有相当大的比重。《难经》对《内经》中所提出的"寸口诊法"(寸口指的是腕部桡动脉搏动所在部位)进行了发展,确立了"独取寸口"的诊脉方法,目前在中医临床中一般都采用"独取寸口"的诊脉方法来诊断病情。《难经》指出由于寸口为"脉之大会",是十二经脉经气汇聚之处,论述了切脉独取寸口能够诊断疾病的原理;又详细指出寸口部位寸、关、尺三部的阴阳属性,每部的浮、中、沉三候,以及与脏腑经络的配合关系,丰富了寸口诊脉的机理;还具体讨论了正常和异常的脉象的不同及其所反映的临床意义。

(1) Elaboration on sphygmology

Compared with *Huangdi's Internal Classic*, *Classic of Difficult Issues* covers quite a lot about sphygmology, which develops "*cunkou* pulse-taking method" in *Huangdi's Internal Classic*(*cunkou* refers to radial artery at the wrist), establishes "taking pulse at *cunkou* alone" method that is still commonly used in clinical practice. The book enriches the mechanism of *cunkou* pulse-taking method as it states that *cunkou* is the place where qi of twelve meridians converges, expounds the principle of this diagnostic method, and contains detailed description of yin-yang properties of three positions (cun, guan, chi) and three pulse conditions (fu, zhong, chen) of each position, as well as relationship among *cunkou*, zang-fu viscera, meridians and collaterals. It also discusses specifically the differences between normal and abnormal pulse conditions and their clinical significance respectively.

(2) 命门的提出

在阐述机体内的脏腑生理功能时,《难经》首次把右肾称为命门,明确了命门与肾的

(2) Proposal of the vital gate (mingmen) (GV4)

On the exposition of physiological function of zang-fu organs, it is *Classic of Difficult Issues* that first calls right kidney the vital gate and makes the distinction between the

关系。如《三十六难》中说："肾两者,非皆肾也。其左者为肾,右者为命门。命门者,诸精神之所舍,元气之所系也。男子以藏精,女子以系胞"。建立了"左肾右命门"的理论,旨在强调人体存在生命之门户,即生命的根本——肾,将肾间动气与命门紧密联系在一起,强调了命门在人体生理活动上的重要作用,从而开创了后世命门学说的先河。

vital gate and kidney. For example, a sentence written in *Thirty-Six Difficult Issues* (*Sanshiliu Nan*) goes that: there are really two kidneys, namely the left one being the actual kidney, while the right being the vital gate, the source of life. The vital gate is the place where essence (*Jing*) gathers and where primordial qi retains. It is also the place where essence is stored for male and where the uterus is nourished for female. *Classic of Difficult Issues* establishes the theory of "left kidney and right the vital gate", aiming to emphasize on the gate of vitality—kidney and the vital gate's important role in physiological activity. The book links interrenal qi closely with the vital gate, carving out the way for the vital gate theory proposed in later ages.

(3) 脏腑的补充

《难经》对人体"三焦"的概念和功能也做了较详细的论述,并记载了五脏六腑的形态,描述了一些脏腑器官的周长、直径、长度、宽度以及重量、容量等,补充了《内经》的人体解剖知识。

(3) Supplement to zang-fu organs

The concept and function of triple energizers (sanjiao) in the body are also introduced in detail in *Classic of Difficult Issues*. It also records the forms of five zang-organs and six fu-organs and describes the perimeter, diameter, length, width, weight and capacity of some zang-fu organs, thus supplementing the knowledge of human anatomy in *Huangdi's Internal Classic*.

(4) 经络学说的补充

《难经》对于《内经》中没有系统阐述的奇经八脉的含义、内容、循行部位、起止、与十二经脉的关系以及发病证候等,都做了较全面的叙述,使经络学说更为完善,并且还着重讨论了针刺补泻法的运用,其中包括了迎随补泻法、补母泻子法、泻火补水法,以及补泻的手法和步骤、误用补泻的不良后果等。这些内容大大丰富了《内经》中所涉及的针刺疗法,而且具有重要的临床指导意义,丰

(4) Supplement exposition to meridian-collateral theory

Classic of Difficult Issues gives a comprehensive exposition to the following aspects of eight extra meridians: the implication and content, the distribution, the starting and ending acupoints, the relationship with twelve meridians and syndrome of diseases, which improves meridian-collateral theory greatly. In the book, the application of strengthening and reducing by needling is also emphatically discussed, mainly including directional reinforcement and reduction method, mother-tonifying child-reducing method, fire-reducing water-supplementing method, manipulation and steps of reinforcing- reducing methods, negative effects of misusing reinforcing-reducing methods. These content greatly enriches acupuncture therapy mentioned in *Huangdi's Internal Classic* and its clinical treatment scope, therefore

富了临床治疗内容。

has clinical guiding significance.

三 学术价值

《难经》从成书后，就被作为重要的医籍而流传，其中确立的“寸口诊脉法”为后世医家所遵从和采用。《难经》的“独取寸口”法改变了《内经》的全身遍诊法，为后世普遍推行寸口诊脉法奠定了基础，直到现在还指导着中医临床脉诊实践；书中对“命门”、“三焦”和“奇经八脉”等的论述，也为后世医家所承袭。因此历代医家对《难经》颇为重视，注释者也不少，它是继《黄帝内经》之后的又一部中医经典著作。中国著名史学家司马迁曾经评价《难经》说：“天下至今言脉者，由扁鹊；盖论脉莫精于《难经》。”

3 Academic value

After its compilation, *Classic of Difficult Issues* spreads as an important medical work, in which, cunkou diagnostic method is followed and employed by doctors in later generations taking the place of diagnostic method all over the body introduced in *Huangdi's Internal Classic*, laying the foundation for cunkou diagnostic method carried out for generations. This diagnosis guides the TCM clinical practice of pulse-taking until now. The elaborations on the vital gate, triple energizers, eight extra meridians in the book are also inherited by later doctors. So *Classic of Difficult Issues*, as an important medical classic after *Huangdi's Internal Classic* is attached great importance by doctors of all dynasties and many glossarists emerge. Sima Qian, a famous Chinese historian, once remarked: "Among the people who feel the pulse through the ages, Bian Que is unparalleled; for numerous books on pulse, *Classic of Difficult Issues* is second to none".

3 神农本草经(Shennong Bencao Jing)

Shennong's Classic of Materia Medica

一 书籍简介

《神农本草经》,简称《本经》或《本草经》,是我国现存最早的药物学专著。它对战国至东汉时期的用药经验和药物学知识做了系统而全面的总结,不仅为我国药物学的发展奠定了基础,而且极大地促进了临床医学的进步。关于《神农本草经》的成书年代,说法不一:或认为成书于战国时代;或说成书于秦汉时期;还有则说它是神农、黄帝或商周时代的作品;也有人断定成书于东汉时期。"神农"是上古时期的一位部落首领,也是中国古代神话人物,据传神农氏的肚皮是透明的,可以看见各种植物在肚子里的反应,因此他亲尝百草,以辨别药物作用。《神农本草经》的作者并非神农,冠之以"神农"二字,表示对其"尝百草"而知药的尊崇,有尊崇古人而托名的意思。当时人们为了凸显学有根本,多将著作托名古人所著以示重要。这种做法也是一种当时流行的做法,该书并非一人所著,大约是秦汉以来许多医药学家,通过对药物学

1 A brief introduction to the book

Shennong's Classic of Materia Medica (*Shennong Bencao Jing*), which is also called *Classic of Materia Medica* for short, is the earliest classic on materia medica extant in China. The book gives a comprehensive and systematic summary of medication experience and materia medica from Warring States Period to Eastern Han Dynasty, laying a foundation for the development of Chinese materia medica and greatly promoting the progress of clinical medicine. The composition of the book has different versions. Some People believe the text was written in the Warring States Period or in the Qin and Han dynasties. Some argue it was completed during Shennong, Huangdi or the Shang and Zhou dynasties, while some predicate the book was compiled in the Eastern Han Dynasty. Shengnong, one of the tribal rulers in prehistoric China, is also a mythological figure. It is told that he tasted hundreds of herbs to test their medical effect, since the reactions of plants can be seen in his transparent belly. In fact, the author of *Shennong's Classic of Materia Medica* is not Shennong. Personally tasting hundreds of medical herbs to test their properties, he was venerated by people. The book entitled with his name could highlight the solid foundation of the study and reflect its value and authority. This practice was quite common at that time. More than one person wrote the book. It is speculated that the book was compiled by many medical experts through keeping on collecting data on pharmacology

资料的不断搜集整理而编写成。"本草"一词是药物的代名词,因为古代所使用的药物以草本药物为主,故用"本草"指药物。

since the Qin and Han dynasties. The word "Bencao" is synonymous with medicine. In the ancient times, herbs and plants were the most frequently-used materials, that's why medicine was called Chinese materia medica.

二 主要内容

全书共收载药物三百六十五种,其中植物药二百五十二种,动物药六十七种,矿物药四十六种。这些药物大多疗效确实,被沿用至今。如麻黄平喘,猪苓利尿,黄芩清热等。

2 The main content

The book includes 365 medicines, among which 252 are herbs, 67 are from animals, and 46 are minerals. Most of these medicines are effective and practical till now. For example, ephedra(mahuang) can relieve asthma, polyporus (zhuling) can promote diuresis, baical skullcap root (huangqin) can clear heat.

(1) 三品药物分类法

《神农本草经》根据药物性能功效的不同,创立了药物的三品分类法,即把全部药物分为上、中、下三品。上品药一百二十种,一般无毒或毒性较小,是"多服久服不伤人"的,可以作为补养类药物长期服用;中品药一百二十种,或有毒或无毒,"斟酌其宜"而使用的,是具有补养和攻治疾病作用的药物;下品药一百二十五种,有毒的居多,"不可久服",大多为除去身体的寒热、破身体内的积聚等攻治疾病的药物。这是中国药物学史上最早出现的药物分类法。

(1) Three-level classification of medicines

Based on its actions and effects, the medicinals are divided into three classes: superior, common and inferior. 120 superior medicinals are nontoxic or low toxic, indicated for long-term administration to treat disease as tonics. 120 common medicinals are toxic or nontoxic, having the dual action of tonifying the body and dispelling pathogens. 125 inferior medicinals are mainly indicated for expelling pathogens by removing the cold heat and relieving the accumulation in the body, many of them are toxic and prolonged administration is forbidden. This is the earliest medicinal classification method in the history of pharmacology.

(2) 提出君臣佐使、七情合和的药物配伍原则

《神农本草经》在《黄帝内经》"君臣佐使"药物主次配伍原则的基础上,对使用药物组合方剂的理论做了进一步阐述,如提出可以"一君

(2) Proposal of ingredient compatibility based on structure of sovereign, minister, assistant and guide and harmony in seven ways

Based on the primary and secondary principle of compatibility of medicines in *Huangdi's Internal Classic*, *Shennong's Classic of Materia Medica* further elaborates the formula-forming theory with drugs. For example, it puts

二臣五佐”、“一君三臣九佐”来进行君臣佐使的药物配伍；同时提出“七情合和”的学说，即单行、相须、相使、相畏、相恶、相反、相杀七种，其中单行是指用单味药治病，其余六种是属于药物之间配伍的关系，相须、相使配伍的药物可增强药效，相恶关系的药物可降低药效，相反关系的药物会产生毒性或者副作用，相畏相杀的关系是指有毒的药物的毒性减轻或者消除。

forward some representative types of formulation, such as "1-sovereign 2-minister 5-assistant" and "1-sovereign 3-minister 9-assistant". The book also presents the theory of "harmony in seven ways of compatibility", namely single effect, mutual reinforcement, mutual assistance, mutual restraint, mutual inhibition, incompatibility, mutual suppression, which means there are seven emotions and effects among herbs when making up a formula. Single effect means treating the illness with a single medicine while the other six conditions reflect the relationships of compatibility of ingredients. Medicines with mutual reinforcement or mutual assistance can enhance therapeutic effects; medicines with mutual inhibition may reduce effects; medicines of incompatibility may produce toxic and side effects; mutual restraint or mutual suppression means the toxicity of poisonous drugs may be inhibited or relieved.

（3）对药物其他方面的介绍

《神农本草经》指出药物有“酸、咸、甘、苦、辛五味，又有寒、热、温、凉四气，及有毒无毒”的特点，除记录有药物的性能外还叙述了药物的产地、采集时间、加工制作方法，以及药物的真伪辨别等内容；在药物剂型制作方面提出要根据不同的病因病机和正气盛衰的情况制作与之相适应的剂型；尤其说明对于有毒性作用的药物，要特别谨慎，强调必须从小剂量开始，逐渐增加剂量，以免造成药物中毒的严重后果。此外还特别重视药物服用的时间和方法，如“病在胸膈以上者，先食后服药；病在心腹以下者，先服药而后食”，反映出对药物临床使用的丰富经验。

(3) Introduction to other aspects of medicines

According to *Shennong's Classic of Materia Medica*, the Chinese medicinal herbs are characterized by five flavors (sour, salty, sweet, bitter, and pungent), four properties (cold, heat, warm, cool), and toxic or non-toxic characteristics, etc. In addition to the properties and actions of medicines, this book describes their growing area, gathering time, processing method and drug identification. It also proposes that the appropriate type of formulation should be matched to the different situations of etiology, pathogenesis and healthy qi. Particularly, the book explains that the medicine with toxic effect should be taken with caution from small dosage to large in case of severe drug intoxication. Besides, the time and method of drug-taking should be paid more attention to. For patients whose diseases occur above chest and diaphragm, the medicine should be taken after meals, while for diseases below heart and abdomen, the medicine should be taken before meals, which reflects the rich experience in clinical application of drugs.

三 学术价值

《神农本草经》作为我国现存最早的一部药物学著作，系统地总结了东汉以前医药学家和民间的用药经验。书中所记录的药物及其功效，在后世长期的临床实践检验和现代科学的研究中已经证明绝大部分都有可靠的疗效，也是目前临床的常用药物。书中提出的药物学理论和用药原则，大多也是正确而具有相当重要的科学价值；所创立的药物三品分类法，虽然较简单原始，但却开创了药物分类的先河。因此《神农本草经》的出现，不但为我国古代的药物学奠定了基础，而且对后世药物学的发展产生了深远的影响。

3 Academic value

As an earliest extant classic on materia medica, *Shennong's Classic of Materia Medica* gives a systematic summary of experts' medication experience before the Eastern Han Dynasty. Most of the herbs recorded in the book are proved to bear reliable curative effects and to be commonly-used in the long-term clinical practice of later ages and modern scientific researches. The theories of materia medica and medication principles proposed in the book are mostly correct and of important scientific value. The three-level classification of medicinals, though simple and original, becomes a pioneer of medicine categorization. Therefore, the appearance of the book not only lays the foundation of ancient pharmacology, but also exerts a far-reaching impact on the development of pharmacology in later generations.

4 伤寒杂病论(Shanghan Zabing Lun)

Treatise on Cold Damage and Miscellaneous Diseases

一 书籍简介

《伤寒杂病论》约成书于东汉末年(200—210),是中医学史上一部非常重要的著作,其作者是被称为"医圣"的东汉名医张仲景。全书共十六卷,包括伤寒和杂病两部分内容,经后世医家整理后分为《伤寒论》和《金匮要略》两部。该书是作者在《黄帝内经》理论的指导下,总结了东汉以前众多医家和作者的临床经验,以六经理论阐述伤寒疾病,以脏腑理论阐述机体杂病,提出了包括理、法、方、药在内的辨证论治思想,是我国医学在临床方面获得迅速发展的一个重要标志。

1 A brief introduction to the book

Treatise on Cold Damage and Miscellaneous Diseases (*Shanghan Zabing Lun*) is a significant medical masterpiece in the history of Chinese medicine, which was compiled approximately at the end of the Eastern Han Dynasty (200—210A. D.). It was written by Zhang Zhongjing, a well-known physician in the Eastern Han Dynasty, who was regarded as the sage of Chinese medicine. The book consists of 16 volumes, containing two parts—cold damage and miscellaneous diseases. After being organized by later physicians, it was divided into two books, namely *Treatise on Cold Damage* (*Shanghan Lun*) and *Synopsis of Prescriptions of the Golden Chamber* (*Jingui Yaolüe*). Under the guidance of the theory in *Huangdi's Internal Classic*, the author summarized clinical experience of his own and many physicians before the Eastern Han Dynasty, elaborating cold damage and miscellaneous diseases respectively with "six-meridian theory" and "theory of zang-fu organs", and putting forward treatments based on syndrome differentiation including principles, methods, prescriptions and medicines—which symbolized China's rapid development in clinical medicine.

二 主要内容

(1) 确立辨证论治原则

《伤寒杂病论》继承了《黄帝内经》的基本理论,将理论与临床实践紧密结合起来,

2 The main content

(1) Establishing the principle of syndrome differentiation and treatment

Based on the basic theory in *Huangdi's Internal Classic*, *Treatise on Cold Damage and Miscellaneous Diseases* combines

确立了理、法、方、药的辨证论治原则。

theory with clinical practice closely, establishing the principle of syndrome differentiation and treatment which involves principles, methods, prescriptions and medicines.

① 六经论治

六经辨证是《伤寒论》论述人体感受外邪后患外感疾病后的辨证思想，其中概括了机体脏腑、经络、气血的生理功能和病理变化，并根据人体抗病能力的强弱、病因的属性、病势的进展缓急等因素，将外感疾病演变过程中所出现的错综复杂的证候进行分析、综合、归纳，以讨论病变的部位、证候特点、寒热趋向、邪正消长，以及立法处方，从而提出了较完整的六经辨证体系。

① Diagnosis and treatment in accordance with the theory of six meridians

Six-meridian syndrome differentiation is about the thought of differentiation proposed in *Treatise on Cold Damage* when people suffer diseases caused by exogenous pathogenic factors. Physiological function and pathological change of body's zang-fu organs, collaterals and meridians and qi and blood are summarized in this thought. In addition, the book analyzes and concludes complicated syndromes caused by external-contraction diseases according to different factors, such as resistance to disease, nature and tendency of an illness. So a relatively complete system of six-meridian syndrome differentiation is established by discussing the location of disease, syndrome characteristics, tendency of chills and fever, exuberance and debilitation of pathogenic qi or healthy qi, as well as establishing therapies and making up formulas.

② 以病分篇

《金匮要略》主要讨论人体所患的除外感疾病以外的杂病，全书共有二十五篇，采取以病分篇的方法，首篇《脏腑经络先后病》是全书的总论，具有纲领性的意义，对疾病的病因、病机、预防、诊断、治疗有原则性的论述。《金匮要略》以整体观念为指导思想，以脏腑经络学说为基础，认为疾病的产生都是整体功能失调、脏腑经络病理变化的反应，提出“若五脏元真通畅，人即安和”的观点，即人体内脏腑功能正常，相互协调，则

② Dividing chapters according to diseases

Synopsis of Prescriptions of the Golden Chamber gives an account of miscellaneous diseases in addition to external-contraction ones. The book is divided into 25 chapters according to different diseases. The first chapter *Zang-fu and Meridian Change Successively*, as the overview of the whole book, has the guiding significance. In this chapter, etiology and pathogenesis, prevention, diagnosis and treatment are all expounded. Based on the theory of zang-fu organs and meridians and taking the holistic concept as guiding ideology, it holds that diseases all result from overall dysfunction and pathological changes of zang-fu organs and meridians. Besides, it puts forward that "if primordial qi performs well in five-zang organs, people will live in a healthy and harmonious way", which means people would rarely get sick with normal function and intercoordination of body viscera. As to the treatment, there

人不容易生病。在治疗中《金匮要略》非常强调有病早治和防止疾病传变发展的观点，如提出"见肝之病，知肝传脾"的认识。同时书中还对病因认识提出了最早的三因致病说，为中医病因学说奠定了基础。

is a very strong emphasis on the early treatment and prevention of the development of diseases. For example, it considers that "the doctor should know the malfunction of liver will transmit to spleen while treating hepatopathy". On the etiology, it also puts forward the earliest theory of three categories of disease causes, which lays a foundation for etiology of Chinese medicine.

(2) 对方剂学的贡献

《伤寒杂病论》共有方剂375首，其中《伤寒论》113首，《金匮要略》262首。除去重复的方剂，实际有269首，基本概括了临床各科的常用方剂。这些方剂立方严谨，用药精炼，绝大多数都行之有效而流传至今，其中不少仍是目前临床的常用方剂，因此该书也被誉为"医方之祖"。

(2) The contribution to Chinese medical formulas

Treatise on Cold Damage and Miscellaneous Damage includes 375 formulas in total, in which 113 are included in *Treatise on Cold Damage* and 262 in *Synopsis of Prescriptions of the Golden Chamber*. Except for repetitive formulas, there are 269 in fact, almost covering commonly-used clinical formulas in various departments. As these formulas are rigorous and pharmaceutically refined, most of them are effective and handed down to generations. At present, many formulas among them are still widely applied in clinical practice. Therefore, the book has been hailed as "the father of the formulas".

书中还非常注重药物的炮制和剂型，记载了炙、熬、煮、酒洗等多种炮制方法，提出通过炮制药物而改变药物性质，以增强药物作用或减轻药物毒副作用，还针对患者的不同病情需要采用不同的药物剂型，如汤剂吸收快药力大，奏效显著，能随症加减，适合复杂临床变化的特点，故应用最为广泛；丸剂药性舒缓，尤适用久病不能速效者；散剂奏效较汤剂更为迅速，且无须煎煮，服用便利，在抢救危急病人时可首选，并创制了外治

Paying attention to processing of materia medica and dosage forms, the book records many processing methods, such as stir-frying with liquid adjuvant, boiling, decocting and washing with spirit. It points out that the nature of drugs can be changed by processing in order to enhance the effects or relieve the toxic and side effects. According to different situations of disease, doctors should choose different dosage forms. For example, decoction is most widely applied for its suitability to complex clinical changes as it can be assimilated quickly with efficacy and modified in accordance with symptoms, while round pills with moderate properties are especially indicated for prolonged illness. Powder, quicker than decoction in effect, needn't to be decocted and can be taken conveniently, therefore, it is the first choice in rescuing critical patients. Meanwhile, some forms for external therapy are created, for example,

法的剂型，如用于治疗便秘塞入肛门的蜜煎导，用作洗剂治疗皮肤病的苦参汤等。书中所记载的包括汤剂、散剂、酒剂、洗剂、熏剂，栓剂、滴耳剂、灌肠剂、含化剂以及软膏等多种剂型已远远超过以往书籍和简帛的内容。

Honey Suppository—which is used to treat constipation by stuffing into anus, and Radix Sophorae Flavescentis Soup (*Kushen Tang*), which serves as a lotion in the treatment of skin diseases. The various dosage forms recorded in the book, such as decoction, powder, vinum, lotion, fumigant, suppository, eardrops, enema, sucking dosage and ointment, are far richer than the content of the previous books and bamboo-silk documents.

三 学术价值

《伤寒杂病论》是我国医学史上影响最大的著作之一，故后人把《伤寒论》和《金匮要略》都视为中医的经典著作。从成书以来它所确立的辨证论治原则，始终有效地指导着临床实践。书中所提出的六经辨证、病症结合的辨证方法被后代医家推崇备至，这种辨证论治的思想不仅对后世临床医学的发展做出了重大贡献，而且迄今仍在临床上发挥着作用。历代许多有成就的医学家无一不重视对《伤寒杂病论》的研究，并把它视为习医者的必读之书。后世医家对《伤寒论》和《金匮要略》的研究非常盛行，出现了大量注解、阐发《伤寒论》和《金匮要略》的著作。自唐宋以来，《伤寒杂病论》的影响还远及日本、朝鲜及东南亚各国。

3 Academic value

Treatise on Cold Damage and Miscellaneous Diseases is one of the most significant works in the history of Chinese medical science, so *Treatise on Cold Damage* and *Synopsis of Prescriptions of the Golden Chamber* are both considered as classics on Chinese medicine by later generations. The principle of syndrome differentiation and treatment established in this book have always been effective in clinical practice. Other methods that are highly favored by later physicians, such as six-meridian syndrome differentiation and the combination of disease and syndrome, not only make great contributions to the development of clinical medicine, but also play an effective role in clinic to this day. In the past ages, many medical scientists with achievements all gave priority in studying *Treatise on Cold Damage and Miscellaneous Diseases* and took it as a required book that practitioners must read. Due to further studies by later generations on *Treatise on Cold Damage* and *Synopsis of Prescriptions of the Golden Chamber*, a lot of works which commented on or elucidated the two books were compiled by later doctors. The influence of *Treatise on Cold Damage and Miscellaneous Diseases* has reached as far as Japan, Korea and Southeast Asia since the Tang and Song dynasties.

5 脉经(Mai Jing)

Pulse Classic

一 书籍简介

《脉经》是中国现存最早的脉学专著,成书约在晋朝初年,作者是晋代的王叔和,曾做过太医令(古代官职,指掌管医事行政的官员),据记载其性格沉静,喜好医术,广泛地学习了当时的医学著作。他将古代脉学的文献资料进行了系统化的整理,并且自己在《脉经》一书的序中写明了著书的目的,指出由于脉学的理论深奥不容易理解,使得临床的脉诊方法和技术难以掌握,如果诊脉稍有差错,则会造成对疾病的错误诊断而形成危害。王叔和所著《脉经》可以说是对中国三世纪以前脉学研究的一次总结。

1 A brief introduction to the book

Pulse Classic (*Mai Jing*) is the earliest extant classic on sphygmology in China. It was written in the early Jin Dynasty by Wang Shuhe, who had been Taiyiling (an ancient official position, in charge of medical administrative affairs). It was recorded he was gentle and quiet by nature, studying medical works of the day widely since he was fond of them. Sorting out ancient documents on sphygmology systematically, he specified the purpose of writing this book in the preface of *Pulse Classic*, pointing out that the clinical pulse-taking methods and techniques were hard to grasp mainly because the theory of sphygmology was too abstruse to understand and a slight mistake in pulse-taking would result in error diagnosis, thus doing harm to human body. To some extent, *Pulse Classic* gives a summary of sphygmology researches before 3rd century in China.

二 主要内容

(1) 规范脉象

《脉经》将临床常见的脉象的名称进行了规范化,共归纳为二十四种脉象,这二十四脉虽然在《黄帝内经》里都提到过,但有关的描述较繁杂而零乱,经过王叔和的系统整理,删除和合并了某些类似

2 The main content

(1) To normalize pulse condition

Pulse Classic normalizes the names of clinical common pulse conditions and reduces them to 24 kinds in total. These conditions have been mentioned in *Huangdi's Internal Classic*, but the relevant account is miscellaneous and in disorder. Thanks to Wang Shuhe's systematic arrangement, some similar pulse conditions are deleted and merged.

脉,从而确立了脉象的基本而较明确的概念。书中在每一种脉象下面,对其形状、指下的感觉、与相同脉象的区别,都一一加以说明,便于学习者对各种脉象的认识、掌握和运用,为后世师徒传授诊脉知识和脉诊教学提供了便利。

Consequently, the basic and more explicit concept of pulse condition is established. With regard to each condition, the book explains its shape, feelings of a physician's fingers, and the differences between the similar pulses one by one so as to make learners to understand, master and apply easily, providing convenience for later generations to impart and teach pulse-taking knowledge.

(2) 确立了"独取寸口"诊脉方法的地位

在公元2世纪以前医生的切脉多为遍诊法,即切人体人迎(相当于颈动脉搏动处)、寸口(相当于腕部内侧桡动脉搏动处)和趺阳(相当于足背动脉搏动处)三个部位,到东汉末年至晋初时期(约公元2世纪时期),"独取寸口"的诊脉方法十分盛行,这种诊脉方法使得患者和医生都感到比较方便。在《脉经》成书后,基本确立了"独取寸口"诊脉法的地位,从此医生临床诊断就逐渐不再使用人迎、趺阳两个切脉部位了。

(2) To establish the status of pulse-taking diagnosis of "only selecting cunkou"

Before the 2nd century A. D., physicians mostly adopted the general diagnostic method, namely, pulse examination on three portions including Renying (ST9) (where the carotid artery pulsates), cunkou (where the radial artery on medial sides of the wrist pulsates), Fuyang (BL59) (where the dorsalis pedis pulsates). However, from the late Eastern Han Dynasty to the early Jin Dynasty (approximately 2nd century A. D.), cunkou diagnostic method turned to prevail because it was convenient for both physicians and patients. After the compilation of *Pulse Classic*, cunkou diagnostic method was basically established while pulse-taking on Renying and Fuyang were seldom used from then on.

(3) 明确提出左右手六脉分配脏腑的理论

《黄帝内经》书中将医生所切取的脉象按照在手指下的感觉层次分为上、中、下三部,但寸口部位的脉位没有分寸关尺部位的不同;《难经》一书创立了寸口部位的切脉部位为寸、关、尺三部(相当于桡动脉搏动处的远心端、中段和近心端),但还没有后世非常

(3) To put forward definitely the correspondence theory of six pulse conditions of two hands and zang-fu organs

In *Huangdi's Internal Classic*, pulse conditions are divided into three sections (upper, middle and lower) according to different feelings of the physician's fingers while taking pulse, but there is no division of cun, guan, chi at the location of cunkou. *Classic of Difficult Issues* presents that cunkou is divided into three portions, namely *cun*, *guan* and *chi* (the equivalence of the distal, middle and proximal end to heart of pulsative place of the radial

明确的左右手寸、关、尺与人体脏腑对应，直至《脉经》一书才明确提出了左右手的寸关尺六个部位的脉象对应人体脏腑的理论，从此这成为脉诊在临床上诊断脏腑疾病的重要理论依据。

artery), but there is no clear record on *cun*, *guan*, *chi* and their corresponding zang-fu organs. It is *Pulse Classic* that puts forward specifically that six portions of *cun*, *guan* and *chi* on two hands correspond to six zang-fu organs respectively, which provides an important theoretical basis for making clinical diagnosis of zang-fu diseases by pulse-taking methods from then on.

三 学术价值

《脉经》在成书后的一段时间内，由于文字所阐述的道理深奥，未能引起医家们的普遍重视，之后才逐渐被越来越重视，到了唐代该书成为医科学生学习的主要教科书之一。《脉经》自诞生后也流传到了国外，对阿拉伯、日本、朝鲜、越南等国家的脉学的形成和发展产生了深远的影响。后世医家对《脉经》均有高度的评价，几乎把它与《黄帝内经》、《神农本草经》、《伤寒杂病论》等并列，可见它在中医学上的重要作用与地位。

3 Academic value

Due to abstruse principles expounded in the text, *Pulse Classic* did not gain much attention from physicians after its completion. Afterwards, it gradually gained more attention and was taken as one of the main textbooks of medical students in the Tang Dynasty. The book made a profound influence on the establishment and development of sphygmology in Arabia, Japan, Korea and Vietnam since it was spread abroad. Physicians in later generations all set a high value on the book and hold that the book can be bracketed with *Huangdi's Internal Classic*, *Shennong's Classic of Materia Medica*, and *Treatise on Cold Damage and Miscellaneous Diseases*, etc., which fully demonstrates the important role and status of the book in Chinese medicine.

6 针灸甲乙经(Zhenjiu Jiayi Jing)

A-B Classic of Acupuncture and Moxibustion

一 书籍简介

针灸作为秦汉以前临床中最常使用的医学技术,《黄帝内经》和《难经》中已记载了丰富的经验和理论认识,并产生了扁鹊、华佗等针灸大家。《黄帝三部针灸甲乙经》(后被称为《针灸甲乙经》或《甲乙经》)是中国现存最早的针灸学专著,该书大约在256—259年间著成,由晋代的著名医家皇甫谧撰写。皇甫谧自幼家境贫寒,但从青年始即发愤苦读,后终成为"博综百家之言"的大学者,42岁时因患风痹而潜心研究医学,尤其致力于针灸学的研究。在该书的自序中作者说因为当时所见到的《内经》书籍已经有所亡失并且编排次序有乱,内容深奥,理论内容偏多而临床实用技能的篇幅较少,不便于阅读,因此从切合实用和教学传授针灸学术的目的出发而撰写该书。该书是在《黄帝内经》中的《素问》及晋以前形成的针灸著作、有关文献的基础上,吸收《难经》等著作的部分内容以及秦汉以后的针

1 An introduction to the book

As the most frequently used medical technique in clinical application before the Qin and Han dynasties, acupuncture and moxibustion had accumulated rich experience and theoretical knowledge as recorded in *Huangdi's Internal Classic* and *Classic of Difficult Issues*. *A-B Classic of Acupuncture and Moxibustion* (*Zhenjiu Jiayi Jing*) (being called *A-B Classic* later), the earliest extant book on acupuncture and moxibustion, was written by a famous physician—Huangfu Mi in the Jin Dynasty and completed around 256—259 A. D. The author, though born in a poor family, decided to make a firm resolution to learn since he was young and finally became an encyclopedic scholar. He got wandering arthritis in the age of 42 and therefore devoted himself to the study of medical science, especially in acupuncture and moxibustion. In the preface of the book, the author mentioned that it was inconvenient for reading as *Internal Classic* he saw earlier at that time was incomplete and disordered, and its content was too profound in theory while inadequate in clinic. So he decided to write a book for the purpose of being practical both in clinic and for teaching acupuncture and moxibustion. On the basis of *Plain Questions* in *Huangdi's Internal Classic* and monograph and bibliography on acupuncture and moxibustion before the Jin Dynasty, the book was completed by combining partial content of *Classic of Difficult Issues*, accomplishments of acupuncture and moxibustion after the Qin and Han

灸成就,并结合作者自己的临证经验写成的。

dynasties as well as the author's own clinical experience.

二 主要内容

全书共分十二卷128篇,其中包括脏腑、经络、腧穴、病机、诊断、治疗、禁忌等内容。该书重点是卷七至卷十二,为主治各病的穴位、操作要求及方法。书中对取穴法、下针深浅、艾灸壮数及留针时间等都做了详细的介绍。

2 The main content

The book consists of 12 volumes (128 chapters), including zang-fu organs, meridians and collaterals, acupoints, pathogenesis, diagnosis, treatment, contraindications, etc. The essence of the book is from volume 7 to volume 12, covering acupoints that cure various diseases, manipulating standards and techniques. There are also detailed introduction to point selection, depth of insertion, the number of moxa cones in moxibustion and time for needle retention.

(1) 系统整理了人体腧穴

该书参考古医书进行归纳、整理后,共确定腧穴349个,其中双穴300个,单穴49个,较《黄帝内经》所记载的穴位增加了189个。书中对这些穴位均有确定的名称、部位及取穴方法等描述。

(1) Systematic conclusion of human body acupoints

The book confirms 349 acupoints through arrangement of ancient medical books and gives all of them specific descriptions with names, locations and selection methods. Among which, there are 300 dual acupoints and 49 single ones. Compared with *Huangdi's Internal Classic*, 189 more acupoints are recorded in this book.

(2) 提出了分部划线布穴的排列穴位方法

将人体的腧穴,按头、面、项、肩、胸、腹、四肢等体表部位排列,四肢分三阴三阳经排列穴位,比《内经》单纯按经络排列穴位,显得清晰、明确,符合人体经络穴位分布规律,确立了后世针灸穴位基本排列规则。

(2) Putting forward the method of acupoint arrangement according to body parts

Compared with arrangement method of acupoints by meridians in *Huangdi's Internal Classic*, this book arranges different acupoints by separating body parts into head, face, neck, shoulder, chest, stomach and four limbs (four limbs are arranged by three yin meridians and three yang meridians), which is more clear and definite, conforming with distribution regularity of meridian-collateral points. Thus, the basic arrangement rules of acupuncture points in later generations are established.

(3) 阐明针灸操作方法和针灸禁忌

书中很详细地描述了九种针具的形状、长度和作用、

(3) Expounding operational approaches and contraindications on acupuncture and moxibustion

The book describes nine kinds of needles in great detail which have different shapes, lengths, functions, needle

针刺手法及补泻的方法、针刺深度等；强调了临床取穴要准确，并要依据个体和疾病而制定具体的治疗方案；并指出临床要掌握针刺的时机，即临床需清楚患者机体的阴阳气血情况，根据病情施以治疗；并提出了8个禁针穴，禁灸的穴位31个等，不宜深刺的穴位4个。

manipulations, reinforcing-reducing methods and depth of insertion, etc. It is emphasized that point selection must be accurate and treatments should be given according to individual syndromes. It also points out the importance of timing on clinic operation, which means the physician should first check the patient's overall condition, including yin, yang, qi and blood circulation, and then decide the treatment accordingly. There are 8 contraacu-points (points that can not be needled), 31 contramoxi-points (points that are forbidden moxa) and 4 points that are forbidden deep insertion.

(4) 总结临床针灸治疗经验，按病论穴

《甲乙经》的第7至第12卷讨论了内、外、妇、儿等科的多种疾病的病因、病机、证候及腧穴、主治，总结了晋以前的针灸治疗经验。书中依据不同的疾病而使用相应的穴位，针对临床上约200种疾病证候，提出可选用腧穴及治疗方法的内容达500余条。

(4) Summarizing clinical treatment experience of acupuncture and moxibustion and selecting acupoints according to diseases

From volumes 7 to 12, it discusses the etiology, pathogenesis, syndrome, acupoints, indications of various illnesses covering subjects from internal medicine, external medicine, gynecology to pediatrics, summarizing treatment experience of acupuncture and moxibustion before the Jin Dynasty. The book also points out that different diseases connect with corresponding acupoints, so over 500 suggestions on acupoint selection and therapeutic method are put forward in accordance with about 200 syndromes in clinic.

(5) 补充了《内经》诸多内容

该书对《内经》做了补充、修改和发展。如《内经》没有记载手少阴经的穴位，《针灸甲乙经》则记载了人体手少阴经的完整腧穴。《内经》所记载的腧穴，一般只属于某一经，《针灸甲乙经》则记载了“三阴交”等穴位不专属于某一经，而是属于多条经脉所交

(5) Supplementing a lot of content to *Neijing*

A-B Classic of Acupuncture and Moxibustion supplements, modifies and develops *Internal Classic*. For example, *Internal Classic* doesn't mention acupoints of hand-shaoyin meridian while in *A-B Classic of Acupuncture and Moxibustion* we can see the complete record of these points. In general, acupoints in *Internal Classic* belong to only one channel, while *A-B Classic of Acupuncture and Moxibustion* records that the acupoints like Sanyinjiao do not belong to a certain channel but an intersection of many channels. From the

会的穴位。这些都说明到了魏晋时期,人们对经络穴位的认识,较战国和秦汉时期又前进了一步。

above, greater advances have been made on knowledge of meridian acupoints in the Wei and Jin dynasties compared with that in the Period of Warring States and Qin and Han dynasties.

三 学术价值

《针灸甲乙经》理论完备,内容实用,是针灸学的经典文献,为后世针灸学的发展建立了规范,在中国针灸学史上占据着重要的地位,对后世影响也非常大。该书保存了大量的古代医学文献,晋以前亡失的针灸文献诸多精要,多赖此书而保存。唐代将此书作为学习医学的教科书,宋、明及清代的众多针灸著作无不参考遵循《针灸甲乙经》。该书不仅成为中医学宝库中的珍藏,而且由此建立了较完整的针灸理论体系,是我国第一部系统性较强,理论、经验完备的针灸学专书。

3 Academic value

The book, as a classic on acupuncture and moxibustion, complete in theory and practical in content, establishes standards for acupuncture and moxibustion development in later generations, holding an important position in the history of Chinese acupuncture and moxibustion and having profound influence on later generations. It preserves a large quantity of ancient medical documents, especially a great amount of essence of acupuncture and moxibustion lost before the Jin Dynasty. In the Tang Dynasty the book was listed as a textbook of medicine and also served as reference book for a lot of works about acupuncture and moxibustion in the Song, Ming and Qing dynasties. It is considered not only as an enshrinement of traditional Chinese medicine, but also as the first systematic monograph on acupuncture and moxibustion with complete theoretical system and adequate clinical experience.

7 本草经集注(Bencaojing Jizhu)

Collective Commentaries on Classics of Materia Medica

一 书籍简介

自药物学专著《神农本草经》成书以来,到晋代时期临床上新的药物品种逐渐增多,并且经长期的临床实践,发现一些药物的性能和主治部分与原有记载有所不同,因此南北朝时期的著名药物学家陶弘景将《神农本草经》和《名医别录》(此书为魏晋以后有关药学著作的编辑书籍)进行了总结,编撰成《本草经集注》3卷。该书成于公元493—500年之间,可谓继《神农本草经》之后我国药物学的又一次总结。

1 A brief introduction to the book

From the completion of the book on materia medica—*Shennong's Classic of Materia Medica* to the Jin Dynasty (265—420A. D.), medicinal varieties increased gradually in clinical practice. However, with long-term practice, it was found that the properties and indications of some drugs were different from the original records. Therefore, Tao Hongjing, a famous pharmacologist in the Northern and Southern dynasties, summarized the contents of two books, *Shennong's Classic of Materia Medica* and *Miscellaneous Records of Famous Physicians* (*Mingyi Bielu*) (the latter is also a book on materia medica after the Wei and Jin dynasties), and compiled them into 3 volumes in this book. The book was accomplished during 493—500A. D. and viewed as another summary of materia medica after *Shengnong's Classic of Materia Medica*.

二 主要内容

(1) 药物总结

陶弘景将《神农本草经》上、中、下三品365种药物和《名医别录》中365种药物合在一起,重新加以分类编排,共计总结了730种药物。该书共三卷,上卷是药物总论,

2 The main content

(1) Summary of herbal medicines

Putting 365 herbal medicines of three classes (superior, common and inferior) in *Shennong's Classic of Materia Medica* and 365 kinds in *Miscellaneous Records of Famous Physicians* together, Tao Hongjing recategorized these drugs and listed 730 medicinal items in total. The book consists of three volumes. Volume 1 is the overview, volume 2 and volume 3 discuss drugs respectively, which

中卷和下卷为药物各论，分为玉石、草木、虫兽、果、菜、米食、有名未用七类。其中中卷包括玉石、草木两类；下卷为虫兽、果、菜、米食四类及有名未用一类。

can be divided into seven categories—jade and stone, grass and trees, insects and beasts, fruits, vegetables, rice and food, and the unused drugs with names. Volume 2 includes two categories—jade and stone, grass and trees. Volume 3 includes insects and beasts, fruits, vegetables, rice and food, and the unused drugs with names.

(2) 创立新的药物分类方法

药物的分类方法是研究药物学的重要组成部分。陶弘景认为所看到的本草学著作散乱而不够系统和完整，而《神农本草经》的三品药物分类法将药物的寒热之性混杂在一起，草类、石类、虫类和兽类等药缺乏更精确的辨别，不利于临床医生的全面掌握。于是他加以系统地整理和研究，提出了按照药品自然属性分类药物的方法，分为玉石、草木、虫兽、果、菜、米食、有名未用等7类，另外还根据临床用药的需要，创立按药物功能分类的方法，如具体列举了80多种疾病的通用药，治风的通用药有防风、防己等，消水肿的通用药有大戟、甘遂、泽泻等。这种按照药物功能分类的方法十分有利于医生的临床使用。

(2) Establishing new classification method of drugs

Classification of medicinal herbs is an important part of pharmacology research. Tao Hongjing held that the works on materia medica he saw were in disorder, not systematic and incomplete to some extent. And what's more, three-level classification in *Shennong's Classic of Materia Medica* was not conducive for doctors to grasp and differentiate in clinic as it mixed medicines with cold and hot natures together. With his systematic arrangement and research, he put forward a new method classified by natural properties of medicines, according to which, drugs could be divided into seven categories. In addition, another method by drug functions was established according to the needs of clinical medication. For instance, he listed specifically commonly-used drugs of over 80 kinds of diseases, drugs for dispelling wind such as divaricate saposhnikovia root (fangfeng) and fourstamen stephania root (fangji), etc. As well as drugs for eliminating edema including Peking euphorbia (daji), gansui root (gansui), oriental waterplantain rhizome (zexie), etc. This classification method was very beneficial to physicians' clinical practice.

(3) 重视药性的区分

该书还针对药物的性质加以重视和区分，认为药物的寒热属性必须明确，才能在临床

(3) Attaching importance to medicinal properties

The book emphasizes and differentiates the drug properties, holding that the properties must be specified. In this way, drugs can be applied accurately in clinical

上准确使用。因此作者将《神农本草经》所提出的药物“寒热温凉”四种属性又加以具体化，提出了寒、微寒、大寒、平、温、微温、大温、大热等八种。

practice. Therefore, the author further specified four properties of drugs—cold, hot, warm and cool, refining them into eight properties—cold, slightly cold, severely cold, mild, warm, slightly warm, very warm, and very hot.

（4）详叙药物加工炮制和配制法

在药物的加工炮制方面，该书的记载很详细，如对药物有去节、去须、去毛、去枝、抽心、去木心、去壳、去皮、去瓤、擘破、细切、捣碎、熬、煎、煮、蒸等操作方法；还记载了通过对药物的炮制改变药性的具体操作，如用酒洒当归使其保持润的特性，各种虫类药要进行轻微的炒炙等。书中共记录了汤剂、酒剂、散剂、丸剂和膏剂五种剂型。此外《本草经集注》还对药物的产地与疗效关系、药物的形态和鉴别、中毒解救药、服药后的宜忌、不宜入汤酒的药物等都做了新的研究和总结。

(4) Expounding on drug processing and preparation

On drug processing, the book makes a detailed records, which include operational approaches, such as eliminating joints, eliminating tassel, eliminating hair, eliminating branches, taking out cores, eliminating duramen, decladding, removing the peel, removing pulp, split, frittering, pounding to pieces, stewing, frying, boiling, steaming, etc. The book also records specific operations of changing drug properties by processing. For example, spirit can be sprinkled on Chinese angelica (danggui) to keep its moistening property. All kinds of insect medicines should be roasted slightly. The book records 5 dosage forms in total—decoction, vinum, powder, pills, pastes. In addition, the relation between drugs' location and curative effect, drugs' form and identification, toxicide, compatibility and incompatibility of taking drugs, and drugs that unsuited to add to soup and spirit are all researched and summed up anew in *Collective Commentaries on Classics of Materia Medica* (*Bencaojing Jizhu*).

三 学术价值

作者在编纂该书时非常尊重原著，在书写中将《神农本草经》的原文都用红色的墨汁写，将《名医别录》的原文都用黑色的墨汁写，使《神农本草经》和《名医别录》各自的内容不致混淆，从而得以将《神农本草经》的原文保存下来。《本草经集注》在本草学发展史上占

3 Academic value

In compiling the book, the author paid considerable respect to the original work. The text from *Shennong's Classic of Materia Medica* was marked in red ink while the content from *Miscellaneous Records of Famous Physicians* was in black. So the content of the two books was not confused and the original text of *Shennong's Classic of Materia Medica* could be preserved. *Collective Commentaries on Classics of Materia Medica* occupies an important role in the history of

据着重要地位。唐、宋、元、明的许多药物学著作，都受到了它的影响。《本草经集注》所创制的两种分类方法，成为药物学主要的分类法，影响了药物学千余年的发展。

herbalism, which widely influences a lot of works on materia medica in the Tang, Song, Yuan and Ming dynasties. The two classification methods established in the book become the main methods of classifying materia medica, having an impact on the development of materia medica for thousands of years.

8 肘后备急方(Zhouhou Beiji Fang)

Handbook of Prescriptions for Emergency

一 书籍简介

《肘后备急方》(又名《肘后救急方》)一书简称《肘后方》,该书写成于四世纪初。作者是晋代著名的医药学家、道家和博物学家葛洪,他在中国哲学史、医药学史以及科学史上都占有很高的地位。葛洪一生从事了大量的医药实践活动,读了大量的医书.并注重分析与研究。他在行医实践中,善于总结治疗心得和搜集民间医疗经验,并以此为基础,完成了百卷巨著《玉函方》。由于该书的内容比较丰富,难于携带检索,他便将书中有关临床常见病和急病的治疗内容编成《肘后备急方》,使医者能随身携带,有利于应临床急救检索之需要,故此书堪称中医第一部临床急救手册。

1 A brief introduction to the book

Handbook of Prescriptions for Emergency (*Zhouhou Beiji Fang*), which is called *Handbook of Prescriptions* (*Zhouhou Fang*) for short, was completed in the early 4th century. The author, Ge Hong, was a famous physician, Taoist, and naturalist in the Jin Dynasty, who occupies an important position in the history of Chinese philosophy, medicine and science. He devoted his lifetime to extensive medical practice, read a lot of medical books, and laid emphasis on analysis and research. In his medical practice, he was efficient at summarizing treatment experience and collecting folk medical experience. On the basis of this, he compiled a magnum opus of hundreds of volumes— *Medical Books* (*Yuhan Fang*). Because this book was rich in content and not convenient for carrying and retrieval, he recompiled the content on treatment of clinical common diseases and acute diseases into *Handbook of Prescriptions for Emergency*, which could be carried with physicians and was conductive to retrieval of clinical first aid. Therefore the book deserves to be called the first clinical first-aid manual of traditional Chinese medicine.

二 主要内容

(1) 提供了丰富的临床内容

现存的《肘后备急方》共有8卷,其中第1—第4卷(即

2 The main content

(1) Providing rich clinical content

The extant book consists of 8 volumes, among which, internal diseases are recorded in volume 1 to volume 4 (Volume Ⅰ in the original work), such as cardiodynia and

原书的上卷)记载有关内科疾病的内容,如心腹痛、伤寒、中风、咳嗽、发黄等急性病;第5至第6卷(即原书的中卷)记载有关许多外科疾病和五官科疾病的内容,如痈疽、疮疥、耳目咽喉头面等病;第7至第8卷(即原书的下卷)记载其他疾病的内容,如虫兽伤、中毒、百病备急丸散药物和牲畜病等。该书涉及了临床的许多急救内容和传染病、内科、外科、妇科、五官科、精神科、骨伤各科疾病的预防、诊断、治疗等内容。

abdominal pain, typhoid fever, stroke, cough, jaundice and other acute diseases. Volumes 5 to 6 (Volume Ⅱ in the original work) record many surgical diseases and diseases of ophthalmology and otorhinolaryngology, such as ulcer, scabies and treatment of ears, eyes, throats, head and face. Volumes 7 to 8 (Volume Ⅲ in the original work) record other kinds of diseases, such as injury bitten by insects and animals, poisoning, pills and powder for hundreds of emergencies, diseases infected by livestock. The book involves rich content of clinical first-aid and infectious diseases. Besides, it also includes the prevention, diagnosis and treatment of diseases of internal medicine, surgery, gynecology, otolaryngologic department, psychiatry and orthopedics and traumatology.

(2) 提供了大量珍贵的病史资料

该书最早记载了天花病,详细记录了天花发病的表现和预后,是世界上关于天花的最早记载;书中对"沙虱"——东方立克次体引起的恙虫病的描述,也是世界上最早的记载,详细记载了恙虫病的病因、发病表现和预防方法、治疗方法;另外对"尸注"的记载和现代的肺结核十分类似,对其症状和传染的危险性已经有认识;关于"狂犬咬伤"(狂犬病)的论述在中国古代医学文献中也属于最早的记载;葛洪在《肘后方》中首创用狂犬脑组织敷贴在咬伤的创口上,以防治狂犬病的方法。虽然技术上未必会成功,但是葛洪所创方法,具有免疫思想的见解。

(2) Providing a great deal of medical records and data

The earliest record of smallpox with detailed symptoms and prognosis in the world can be found in the book. It also makes an earliest and detailed description of Chigger mites, namely tsutsugamushi caused by rickettsia orientalis, including its cause, onset manifestation, preventive and treatment methods. In addition, the record of "Shizhu" (a corpse attachment-illness that is consumptive and infectious) in the book, as well as certain knowledge of its symptoms and risk of infection, is much similar to tuberculosis in modern times. The exposition on rabies is also the earliest in ancient Chinese medical documents. Ge Hong originated a method for prevention and treatment of rabies in *Handbook of Prescriptions* by applying brain tissue of the infectious dog to the wound, which embodies the insight of immunity though it doesn't necessarily work out technically.

(3) 提供了较多灵活的治疗方法和急救方法

该书对治疗方法的选择不拘一格,提供了临床上可以采用的诸多方法如针灸、推拿、拔罐、蒸、熨等;书中也记录了许多适合急救的简便疗法,如"令爪其病人人中取醒"治疗卒中(急性脑血管疾病)的急救措施至今在民间还常常应用。该书对骨折、脱臼的整复手法和小夹板局部固定法、危重创伤的致死部位及抢救方法,也都一一做了介绍,从而为中医骨伤学形成和发展奠定了基础。在急救方法方面,书中还记载了人工呼吸、止血、腹腔穿刺、导尿、灌肠、清创、引流等急救治疗技术。

(3) Providing quite a lot of flexible therapies and first-aid methods

The book does not stick to one pattern in the choice of therapies, providing many methods which can be used clinically, such as acupuncture, massage, cupping, steaming, compressing, etc. Many simple and convenient methods suitable for first-aid are also recorded in the book. For example, the first-aid treatment of acute stroke (cerebrovascular diseases) by pricking philtrum is commonly used to this day. Reduction of fracture and dislocation, fixed method of body parts with small splints, rescue method and lethal location of critically-wounded patients are introduced separately, thus laying the foundation for TCM formation and development in traumatology and orthopedics. In terms of first-aid methods, many techniques are registered, such as artificial respiration, hemostasis, abdominocentesis, catheterization, enema, debridement and drainage, etc.

(4) 提供了简便验廉的药物

为适应偏僻之地治疗急症的需要,葛洪在书中大力提倡简易有效的治疗办法,所用药物多为山乡易得之物并且价廉、有效,如栀子、葱、姜、豆等,即使在穷乡僻壤求医不方便时,也可自行取方配药。书中还记录了很多简单、方便、有效和廉价的药方,如常山治疟、麻黄治喘、商陆治水肿、大黄治泻下和硫黄、水银等治皮肤病,这些都是古代人民宝贵的用药经验。特别值得指出的是《肘后备急方》中关于青

(4) Providing simple, convenient, effective and inexpensive drugs

In order to meet the needs of emergency treatment, Ge Hong advocates simple and effective treatment in his book. Most of drugs that he applies are usually available even in remote areas, which are cheap and effective, such as cape jasmine, scallion, ginger and bean. Even though in hinterlands, where medical advice is not usually available, people can make up prescriptions and take drugs by themselves. Besides, the book also introduces many therapies with simple, convenient, effective and cheap drugs, such as curing malaria with antifeverile dichroa root (changshan), curing asthma with ephedra, curing edema with pokeberry root (shanglu), curing purgation with rhubarb (dahuang), curing skin diseases with sulfur and mercury, all of which are precious experience of ancient people in using drugs. The most worthy to mention in this

蒿治疟的记载，书中记载了取用山间随处可见的青蒿绞汁饮服，这不仅在当时疗效显著，更为我国现代药理研究提供了宝贵线索，从而在青蒿中提取出高效、速效、低毒的抗疟新药——青蒿素，成为中国医学对世界医学的一项新贡献。带领科研团队发现青蒿素的中国科学家屠呦呦因此获得了2015年诺贝尔生理学或医学奖。

book is the record that malaria can be cured by drinking the extracting juice of sweet wormwood herb (qinghao), which can be seen everywhere in the mountains. This therapy is not only effective in treatment at that time, but also provides valuable clues for modern pharmacological researches in China. On the basis of this, artemisinin (qinghaosu), as a new antimalarial medicine characterized by highly effectiveness, fast-acting and low toxicity, is extracted from sweet wormwood herb, which makes a new contribution to the world's medicine. Together with her team, Tu Youyou, a Chinese scientist who discovered artemisinin and its utility for treating malaria was awarded the Nobel Prize in Physiology or Medicine 2015.

(5) 丰富了灸法的内容

书中记载了很多使用艾条灸治的方法治疗疾病的经验，操作简便，很值得重视。在所记述的72种病中，可以用灸治疗的多达30余种；并且大胆使用灸法治疗急症，如对吐泻腹痛为主的“霍乱”和突然昏烦的“卒中恶死”，均选用承浆穴灸治。同时还最早记载了隔物灸法，详细介绍了隔蒜、隔盐、隔椒、隔面等灸治方法以及蜡灸法等，可谓取材广泛，扭转了晋以前重针刺而忽视灸治的偏颇，丰富了灸疗法的内容，推动了灸治学的发展。

(5) Enriching the content of moxibustion

Rich experience in the treatment with moxa is recorded in the book. They are easy to handle and worth taking seriously. Among the recorded 72 diseases, there are over 30 diseases that can be cured with moxibustion therapy. Especially, moxibustion can be applied to treat emergencies, for example, moxibustion on Chengjiang (CV 24) can treat both sudden stroke and cholera with vomiting, diarrhoea and stomachache. At the same time, many indirect moxibustion therapies are introduced first time in the book, covering a wide range of content such as moxibustion with garlic, salt, pepper, flour and wax, etc. These therapies reverse the situation that caring acupuncture more than moxibustion before the Jin Dynasty, enriching the content of moxibustion therapy and promoting the development of moxibustion.

三 学术价值

葛洪一生以从事医疗实践活动为主，足迹广泛，常走行于民间，并广泛收集民间经验，基于药物方剂的使用要实用有效可靠并且简便易行，即

3 Academic value

Ge Hong has been engaged in medical practice throughout his lifetime, leaving his footprints all over the land and recording folk experience widely. The book is based on effective, practical, reliable and easy-operating usage of prescriptions, which means it is compiled with the

"方药不在于广而在于精，疗法不在于多而在于有效"的思想而编纂成该书，该书问世后，书中许多内容已为后世临床及科学实验证实确实有效，在中国医学史上具有相当的科学价值。

thought that "prescription lies in accuracy rather than variety while therapy rests with effectiveness rather than quantity". After the publication of the book, a lot of content in it has proved to be effective through clinical and scientific researches of later generations, which is of certain scientific value in the history of Chinese medicine.

9 雷公炮炙论(Leigong Paozhi Lun)

Master Lei's Discourse on Medicinal Processing

一 书籍简介

传统中药的使用,常常需要经过加工处理后才运用于临床,这一过程即为中医的药物炮制过程。药物经过炮制后可以除去杂质,或者便于贮存,或者去除、减少药物的毒性,或者改变药物的性质,或者提高药物的药效等。中医关于药物炮制的第一部专书是《雷公炮炙论》。书名中的"雷公"有两种解释,一说是指黄帝时期的大臣,一说是指南北朝时期的雷敩,一般以后者说法为正确。该书实际上是雷敩对药物炮制加工的经验整理,书中总结了大量药物的各种炮制方法,为中药的炮制研究提供了宝贵的资料,奠定了中药炮制学的基础。

1 A brief introduction to the book

Processing of the Chinese materia medica refers to the necessary processes of preparing raw materials before their application clinically. It aims to remove impurities, facilitate storing, eliminate or minimize the toxicity, change the properties, or increase the efficacy, etc. *Master Lei's Discourse on Medicinal Processing* (*Leigong Paozhi Lun*) is the first monograph on the processing of drugs. There are two explanations for the name "Lei Gong" in the title. One goes that he is a minister in Huangdi's period. Another is that Lei Gong refers to Lei Xiao in the Northern and Southern dynasties. It is generally acknowledged the latter is convincible. Actually, the book is the rearrangement of TCM processing by Lei Xiao. The summary of medicinal processing methods in the book provides precious materials for TCM processing research and lays the foundation of TCM processing theory.

二 主要内容

该书共分上、中、下3卷,载药300种,总结了182种药物的各种各样炮制法,如蒸、煮、炒(多为拌合其他物)、焙(微温干燥)、炙(蜜炙、酥炙)、煅(在火中烧红)、浸、水

2 The main content

The book consists of three volumes, which includes 300 drugs. It summarizes various processing methods of 182 drugs, ranging from steaming, boiling, stirring-baking (mostly mixing other materials), baking (to dry medicinal materials with slow fire), stir-baking with liquid adjuvant (such as stir-baking with honey or butter) to calcining (to heat medicinal materials with strong fire), dipping, grinding

飞(加水研末)、制膏(生药煎煮的汁熬成膏浓缩)等,这些丰富的炮制方法促进了中药炮制的发展。

with water (to grind medicinal herb into fine powder in water), ointment making (herb concentration through frying and boiling) and so on. These rich processing methods promote the development of TCM processing.

(1) 减轻药物毒性,增强药物疗效

中药中不少药物都具有一定的毒性,人体直接服用后会有较大的身体伤害,如巴豆这味药有剧毒,书中记载了巴豆的炮制方法,"敲碎,以麻油酒等煮,研膏后用",用油煮后,巴豆中的有效成分——巴豆油可溶解于油,而其毒性蛋白(能溶解红细胞,使组织坏死)则被破坏,这种处理方法可很好地保留巴豆的药物有效成分而降低药物的毒性。

(1) To minimize the drug toxicity and enhance its efficacy

A lot of Chinese materia medica are somewhat toxic and do harm to human body if taken directly. Croton fruit (badou), for example, as recorded in the book, is extremely toxic. It is firstly processed by smashing, then boiling it with sesame oil and spirit, grinding it and making it into plaster afterwards. In this way, its effective compositions are dissoluble to oil and its toxic protein, which can dissolve red blood cells and kill tissues, is destroyed. This processing method can retain its effective medicinal composition and reduce its toxicity.

(2) 保持药物质量,易于保存放置

为了有利于中药的长久保存,书中介绍了多种炮制方法,如经过蒸、煮、炙等加热处理后,药物中的酶素被破坏后就易于保存;像大黄经过切细蒸晒后可较长时间存放,现代研究证实这种处理方法可以防止大黄的有效成分蒽醌甙被酶分解而延长贮存期。书中还指出了对药物的保存注意禁忌,如指出茵陈、槟榔等"勿近火",可减少它们所含挥发油的损失;知母、茜草等忌用铁器,可以防止药物中所含单宁碱素等成分与铁反应;蛇类药用酒浸后能防腐等。

(2) To maintain high quality and facilitate storing

For long-term preservation, the book introduces many processing methods. For instance, medicinals are easily preserved when enzymes are destroyed by some heating methods, such as steaming, boiling, and stir-baking with liquid adjuvant. Dissected rhubarb after steaming and drying in the sun can be preserved for a long time. Latest research proves that this processing method can prevent anthraquinone glycoside (effective constituent of rhubarb) from decomposing by enzymes, so as to extend preservation. Attentions and prohibitions on medicinal preservation are also pointed out. For example, virgate wormwood herb (yinchen) and areca nut (binglang) should keep away from the fire so as to reduce the loss of their essential oil; common anemarrhena rhizome (zhimu) and madder (qiancao) should not be decocted in iron utensils so as to avoid chemical reaction between tannin in the drugs and iron. Medicines made from snake can be antiseptic if soaked with spirit.

（3）提供了丰富的炮制方法

该书在前人经验的基础之上，增添了多种炮制方法，并且每一类炮制大法又有许多不同的处理方法。如浸法根据溶媒的不同性质，分为水浸、盐水浸、蜜水浸、浆水浸、药汁浸、米泔汁浸、酒浸、醋浸等；煮法分水煮、盐水煮、浆水煮、甘草水煮、米泔水煮、药汁煮等。蒸法分为一般蒸、酒拌蒸、黄精汁浸后蒸、生地黄拌蒸以及其他药汁拌蒸等。

(3) To provide abundant processing methods of materia medica

On the basis of former experience, the book adds various processing methods with different procedures. According to different properties of solvent, the procedures of soaking are classified into soaking with water, salt solution, honey water, seriflux, drug juice, rice-washing water, spirit, vinegar and so on. The procedures of boiling include boiling with water, salt water, honey water, seriflux, liquorice water, rice-washing water and drug juice, etc. The method of steaming includes traditional steaming and steaming with spirit, soaked sealwort juice, unprocessed rehmannia root (shengdihuang) and other decoctions.

三 学术价值

中药炮制理论与技术的发展，是中药学发展的重要组成部分。许多传统的中药炮制法是科学的。如果不"如法炮制"，会降低质量，影响疗效。《黄帝内经》和《伤寒杂病论》也有关于某些药物炮制的记载，《雷公炮炙论》是在之前的医学基础上总结经验，加以归纳，形成了系统的中药传统炮制理论和方法。原书早已佚失，现仅存后世从各种有关药物的著作中编辑而成的辑本流传。该书作为一部专门记述药物的性味、煮熬、炮制、修治等理论和方法的专著，较系统地总结了公元5世纪前中药炮制的经验，2000多年来一直受到制药业的高度重视，故此雷敩也被认为是中医药炮制的鼻祖。

3 Academic value

The development of processing theory and technique is an important part of the development of TCM. Many traditional Chinese medicinal processing methods are scientific. If not preparing herbal medicinal by the prescribed method, the quality will be degraded and curative effect will be affected. *Huangdi's Internal Classic* and *Treatise on Cold Damage and Miscellaneous Diseases* also record some processing methods of materia medica. Based on former medical science, the book sums up experience and establishes systematic TCM processing theory and methods. The original book is lost while the only existing version is compiled on the basis of records in various materia medica works. As a monograph recording theories and methods regarding nature and flavor, boiling, processing of materia medica, the book gives a systemic conclusion of processing experience before the 5th century B. C. It has been attached great importance by the pharmaceutical industry for over 2000 years, therefore the author, Lei Xiao, is considered the founder of TCM processing.

10 诸病源候论(Zhubing Yuanhou Lun)

Treatise on the Pathogenesis and Manifestations of All Diseases

一 书籍简介

《诸病源候论》一书是我国现存最早的病源证候学专著,是一部系统论述临床各科疾病的病因病机和症状体征的理论性专著。该书是在公元610年由隋朝政府组织,隋朝太医院的博士巢元方主持编撰而成的,该书也被后人称为《巢氏病源》。巢元方具体的生卒年月不详,在公元605—616期间曾任隋朝太医院的博士,后来担任太医令(古代官职,指掌管医事行政的官员),具有丰富的临床经验,有关史书资料曾记载其临床治病疗效极佳。《诸病源候论·序》中说到该书的编撰宗旨是遵循"医之作也,求百病之本,而善则能全"的精神,即探究疾病的形成之根本,找出病因病源。从《黄帝内经》以来,中医学的发展也都致力于探求疾病的病因病源,并积累了丰富的临床观察经验和认识,该书将医学对病因病源的认识汇集总结,并结合当时医疗实践中的新发现新探索,对

1 A brief introduction to the book

Treatise on the Pathogenesis and Manifestations of All Diseases (*Zhubing Yuanhou Lun*), the earliest extant monograph on pathogenesis and manifestations of diseases, gives a theoretical and systematic exposition on etiology and pathogenesis, symptoms and signs of various clinical diseases. The book, also known as *Chao's Treatise on the Pathogenesis and Manifestations of Diseases* (*Chaoshi Bingyuan*), was organized by the government of the Sui Dynasty in 610 A. D. and compiled by Chao Yuanfang, an imperial court physician whose date of birth and death was unknown. After holding a post as a doctor in the Imperial Academy of Medicine during 605—616 A. D. and later the master of imperial medical affairs (an ancient official who was in charge of medical administrative affairs), the author had accumulated rich clinical experience and the curative effect was excellent as recorded in some relevant historical materials. The preface mentioned that " the book aims to seek the root of all diseases, so as to find the causes to cure them". Since the publication of *Huangdi's Internal Classic*, the development of traditional medicine had been focused on the causes of diseases and accumulated rich experience based on clinical observation and knowledge. The book was not only a conclusion of medical cognition on the causes of diseases but also the elaboration and research on the etiology of clinical diseases or syndromes based on the latest

临床疾病或证候的病因病源逐个进行阐述和研究。

discoveries and exploration on medical practice at that time.

二 主要内容

《诸病源候论》主要是对魏晋时期(约公元2—5世纪)以来医学研究中关于疾病病因来源和病的证候总结汇集，全书共分50卷，包括67门，论述了1739条病候，广泛记载了临床各科疾病。其中卷1至卷27记载风病、虚劳、伤寒、温病、时行以及杂病等内科疾病，分别记载风病59种，记载虚劳75种，其他如消渴、脚气、黄疸、水肿、虫症等也设专章论述；卷28至卷36记载外科、五官、口腔等疾病，其中外科仅金创一类就记载23种病候，又详细论述丹毒、破伤风、结核性疾患、痈疽、痔瘘、火伤、湿疹、疥疮等疾病；记载了眼科病38种，包括青光眼、夜盲症等病症；对五官科疾病如鼻息肉、兔唇等也都有详细记载；卷37至卷44记载妇产科杂病和胎产等疾病，其中妇产科病收载有140多种，详细分为妇人杂病、妊娠病、将产病、难产病、产后病5类，包括月经不调、白带、阴挺、乳痈、妊娠恶阻、难产、产后恶露等多种病症；卷45至卷50着重讨论小儿科杂病及传染病等。

2 The main content

Treatise on the Pathogenesis and Manifestations of All Diseases is a summary and collection on the pathogenesis and manifestations of diseases in medical research during the 2nd—5th centuries (Wei and Jin dynasties). The book consists of 50 volumes and 67 categories, including 1739 syndromes with wide range of clinical diseases. Among which, volumes 1 to 27 describe internal diseases such as wind-evil diseases (59 syndromes), consumptive diseases (75 syndromes), cold damage, warm diseases, seasonal epidemic and other miscellaneous diseases. Other diseases like diabetes, beriberi, jaundice, edema, parasitosis are also discussed in special volumes. Volumes 28 to 36 cover diseases of surgery, five sense organs and stomatology, in which 23 syndromes due to metal-inflicted wound are included. In addition, detailed description on erysipelas, tetanus, tuberculosis, carbuncle, anal fistula, burn, eczema, scabies are also made in this part. There are 38 syndromes of oculopathy, including glaucoma and nyctalopia. Some diseases of five sense organs including rhinopolypus and harelip are also recorded in detail. Volumes 37 to 44 introduce more than 140 syndromes of miscellaneous diseases in the department of obstetrics and gynecology, which are classified into 5 categories as follows: women disease, pregnancy disease, prenatal disease, difficult labor and puerperal disease, and include various syndromes such as irregular menstruation, leucorrhea, prolapse of uterus, acute mastitis, pernicious vomiting with pregnancy, dystocia, postpartum lochia and so on. Volumes 45 to 50 focus on pediatric and contagious diseases.

（1）对许多疾病的病因病源提出正确认识

《诸病源候论》的“疫疠病候”提出传染病是由被称为“乖戾之气”的外界有害物质所引起，并且“生病者多相染易，故须预服药及为方以制之”，即指出传染病的容易传染特性，需要预先服药来防治患病，相比较隋代以前多把流行性传染病列于伤寒、温病中，认为是由于气候变化异常所导致的观点更准确，这些观点对于传染病的认识具有重要意义。对寄生虫病的认识也有深入的了解，能够准确描述病源，如“蛔虫候”说：“蛔虫者……长一尺，亦有长五六寸，或因脏腑虚弱而动，或因食甘肥而动，其发动则腹中痛，发作肿聚，去来上下……，口喜吐涎及吐清水”；其他如对蛲虫、绦虫等皆有虫体形态细致观察，指出蛲虫与脏腑虚弱有关，绦虫与食入生牛肉、鱼肉有关；对恙虫病也准确描述其证候特点和传染途径，如在“沙虱候”中记载：“山内水间有沙虱，其虫甚细不可见，入水浴及汲水澡浴，此虫著身，及阴雨日行草间亦著人”等。在“水毒候”中就血吸虫病源做了一定的论述，指出血吸虫病流行地区是“有山谷溪源处，有水毒病，春秋辄得”。

（1）Correcting misunderstanding on etiology

The volume of *Syndromes of Pestilence* in the book points out contagious diseases are caused by poisonous materials called “evil qi” and “patients are easily infected by each other, so drugs and prescriptions are indispensable for treatment”. The viewpoint is more accurate than what has been held before the Sui Dynasty, that is, the contagious disease belongs to cold damage and warm disease and is caused by abnormal climate change. These points of view are important in exploring the causes of contagious diseases. As regards parasitic diseases, the book also has a deep understanding and gives an exact description about the causes. For instance, *Syndromes of Ascariasis* expounds the length of ascarids ranging from 5 or 6 cun to 1 chi（nearly 20 cm to 30 cm）and they move around either because viscera weakness or eating too much fat. When ascarids move around, the patient may incur the following symptoms such as stomachache, abdominal distension and spitting saliva, etc. Other descriptions like the form of pinworm and tapeworm are quite specific: enterobiasis is linked with weakness of internal organs and teniasis is due to eating raw beef or fish. In terms of tsutsugamushi disease, the features of its syndromes and route of infection are also described clearly. For example, as to chigger, it is recorded that this bug inhabits in mountain and river and is too small to be visible to the naked eye, crawling onto human body when people bath in river or walk in grass in rainy days. The part of *Syndromes of Bilharziasis* expounds the risk of infection is highest among places in valley and near rivers, especially in spring and fall.

(2) 准确描述了许多疾病的临床表现症状

书中汇集临床长期观察经验，对多种疾病临床表现均做了详细而准确的描述，为医生辨识各种疾病提供了可靠依据。如在"诸癞候"中记载麻风病早期为"初觉皮肤不仁，或淫淫苦痒如虫行，或眼前见物如垂丝"；潜伏期则"入皮肤里，不能自觉，或流通四肢，滞于经脉"，其表现"或在面目，或在胸颈，状如虫行，身体遍痒，搔之生疮，或身面肿，痛彻骨髓"，晚期则出现"眉睫堕落"、"鼻柱崩倒"、"肢节堕落"等表现。在"消渴候"中能准确描述消渴病的临床特点如"夫消渴者，渴不止，小便多是"、"其病多发痈疽"，这些都与现代医学对糖尿病认识相吻合。此外书中还对脚气病、中风、黄疸等疾病的临床表现都进行了详细描述，反映出当时医学对这些疾病的研究水平，同时还对很多相似重症进行了鉴别，如区分了热痢与冷痢不同，对天花与麻疹做出了世界医学史上最早的鉴别诊断。

(2) Accurately describing many clinical symptoms

The long-term observation and detailed description on clinical symptoms of various diseases in the book provide reliable basis for illness identification. In *Syndromes of Leprosy*, there is description about symptoms of gafeira in different stages. In the early stage, skin feels numb. Sometimes it tickles like there are worms crawling on it, and sometimes the vision blurs like there is a curtain in front. In the incubation period, patients suffer loss of sensation. The virus circulates into four limbs and stagnates in channels. Symptoms are manifested either in the face, chest or neck, like a sinuous worm crawling and the whole body feels itchy. Sore will appear, body and face will swell up and unbearable pain will incur after scratching. In later period, leprosy will cause body parts to fall off, including eyebrows, eyelashes, nose bridge and four limbs. The clinical syndromes of diabetes, characterized by frequent drinking, micturition and complication of ulcer, are all in accordance with modern cognition on diabetes. Besides, there are also detailed descriptions on the clinical symptoms of beriberi, stroke, and jaundice, etc., which reflect the level of medical research at that time. Meanwhile, the differentiation of many similar severe diseases is made, such as warm diarrhea and cold diarrhea, among which, the differential diagnosis between smallpox and measles appears to be the earliest around the world.

(3) 对创伤性疾病的认识和外科手术的记录

书中对多种创伤性感染的病源和途径作了精辟的描述，如指出破伤风或是与金疮感染有关，在妇人与产褥感染有关，在小儿与脐疮感染有关，并将破伤风与中风等病鉴

(3) Understanding of traumatic diseases and records of surgery

The book gives a penetrating description on causes and transmission of a variety of traumatic infection. For example, it points out that tetanus probably is related to metal-inflicted wound, puerperal infection and baby-umbilical sore infection.

别。书中还记录了不少有关治疗创伤的外科手术方法和缝合技术，如“金疮断肠候”中的肠吻合手术、血管结扎术、创伤异物清除术等；在“妊娠欲去胎候”中记载了人工流产术，“拔齿损候”中记载了拔齿术，在“阴中生息肉候”记载了妇科检查术等，这些都反映了公元7世纪临床医学的新成就。

It also makes a differentiation between tetanus and stroke as well as other diseases. Quite a lot of surgery methods and suture skills are recorded in different volumes, such as intestinal anastomosis, vessel ligation, evacuation of foreign body, artificial abortion, extraction of teeth, gynecologic examination, and so on, all of which represent the new achievements in clinical medicine in 7th century.

（4）发现了某些过敏性疾病

书中“漆疮候”中指出漆疮（即因为接触漆而导致的皮肤过敏）与人的身体禀性有关，并通过“有人接触漆会生病，而有人终日煮漆接触亦不会被影响”相关描述和细微观察，明确肯定这属于过敏性疾病。这些关于过敏性反应的病因归结于个体体质不同的观点，已超出传统的中医病因理论认识范围。

(4) Finding some allergic diseases

The volume of *Dermatitis Rhus Syndromes* points out that dermatitis rhus (skin allergy due to contacting lacquer) is connected with the constitution of human body. By subtle observation and the description that "someone who contacts lacquer will be sick, while others are not affected even in touch with lacquer all day long", the author clearly affirms that lacquer dermatitis is an allergic disease. The view that the etiology of allergic reaction is ascribed to different individual constitution has gone beyond the scope of traditional cognition on Chinese medical etiology.

三 学术价值

《诸病源候论》在疾病的病因理论方面提出很多新见解，有不少创造性的阐述，突破了前人笼统的三因致病（内因、外因和不内外因）理论，丰富了祖国医学的病因学说。这是隋代一部很有价值的医学著作，它对后世的病因证候学有深远的影响，后世不少医学著作都直接或间接地引用书中原文和论点，唐宋以后该书长期成为医学教科书，也是医学生考试的科目之一。

3 Academic value

Treatise on the Pathogenesis and Manifestations of All Diseases puts forward many new ideas in etiology theories, breaking through the indistinct "theory of three categories of disease causes" (internal cause, external cause and cause neither internal nor external) of previous generations, enriching the theory of medical etiology in China. As a valuable medical work in the Sui Dynasty, it exerted a profound impact on etiology and symptomatology of later ages. Many medical works of later generations, directly or indirectly, cited its original text and arguments. After the Tang and Song dynasties, the book has become a medical textbook for a long time and also one of the subjects of medical examination for students.

11 千金方(Qianjin Fang)

Thousand Golden Prescriptions

一 书籍简介

《千金方》是《备急千金要方》和《千金翼方》的简称，作者是唐朝的孙思邈（公元581—682）。孙思邈是中医史上非常重要的医家，因自幼多病，曾耗尽家里的钱财治疗疾病。于18岁时立志学医，终生勤奋攻读医书，也博览群书，精于研究中国历史上的诸多哲学思想，如诸子百家、老庄、佛家经典等，知识渊博。史料记载他曾被皇帝下诏授以爵位，但推辞没有接受，而一生坚持在民间行医。《备急千金要方》写成于其70岁之前，《千金翼方》则为后来所作，是对《备急千金要方》的补充。《千金方》详尽地记载了唐以前主要医学著作的医论、医方、诊法、治法、食养、导引等多方面的内容，包含了作为一个医生所必备的各种医学理论和实践知识，堪称我国第一部医学百科全书。

1 A brief introduction to the book

Thousand Golden Prescriptions (*Qianjin Fang*) is short for *Essential Prescriptions Worth a Thousand Gold for Emergencies* (*Beiji Qianjin Yaofang*) and *Supplement to Essential Prescriptions Worth a Thousand Gold for Emergencies* (*Qianjin Yifang*). The author is Sun Simiao (581—682 A. D.) of the Tang Dynasty, who is a very important doctor in the history of Chinese medicine. In his childhood, he was weak and frequently suffered from illnesses. His disease had cost all his family fortunes, so he was determined to be a doctor at the age of 18. Sun Simiao devoted himself into reading books not only on medical science but on all sorts throughout his life. He had a wide range of knowledge, specializing in research on numerous philosophical thoughts, such as hundreds of various schools, Lao Zi and Zhuang Zi, Buddhist classics and so on. It was recorded that Sun was offered at least three official court positions by the emperor, but he turned down, preferring to treat for folk people all his life. *Essential Prescriptions Worth a Thousand Gold for Emergencies* was completed by him before the age of 70 while *Supplement to Essential Prescriptions Worth a Thousand Gold for Emergencies* was finished later, which replenished the former. *Thousand Golden Prescriptions* deserves to be the first medical encyclopedia in China because what it records covers a lot of content in medical works before the Tang Dynasty in detail, including theories of Chinese medicine, medical prescriptions, diagnostic methods, therapeutic methods, dietary regimen and *Daoyin* (physical and breathing exercises), etc, which involves essential medical theories and practical knowledge for a doctor.

二 主要内容

《备急千金要方》和《千金翼方》各有30卷。《备急千金要方》中包括了总论、妇科病、儿科病、五官科病、内科病、养生、导引、按摩、脉诊、针灸疗法等内容，全书共有方4 500首。《千金翼方》是《备急千金要方》的续编，包括了药物、妇产科病、伤寒病、小儿病、养生补益、中风、杂病、疮痈、诊脉、针灸、祝由等内容。两部书的内容特点可概括为：

(1) 经验丰富 内容实用

两部书的内容极其丰富，总结了内外妇儿各科疾病的治疗以及诊法、针灸、药物知识、养生和食养等大量经验。书中内容集唐朝以前医方之大成，共计6 500余首医方，既有前代著名医家的用方，又有各地民间百姓的验方，还有少数民族医方和国外所传的医方。书中的很多医方流传后世而成为现代医生常用的名方，如清热凉血的"犀角地黄汤"、温阳攻下积滞的"温脾汤"、补气血祛风湿的"独活寄生汤"等，为方剂学的发展做出了贡献。在临床治疗中孙思邈强调综合治疗，不仅主张针药并用，并且创制了彩色经络图，还常配合按摩、艾灸治疗各种疾病，同时他还是食治

2 The main content

Essential Prescriptions Worth a Thousand Gold for Emergencies and *Supplement to Essential Prescriptions Worth a Thousand Gold for Emergencies* are both 30-volume works on medical practice. The former lists about 4,500 prescriptions, covering overview, gynaecology, pediatrics, ophthalmology and otorhinolaryngology, internal medicine, health maintenance, *Daoyin*, massage, sphygmology, acupuncture and moxibustion, etc. The latter is a continuation of the former, including drugs, gynecologic and obstetric diseases, typhoid diseases, infantile diseases, health maintenance and tonifying, stroke, miscellaneous diseases, carbuncle, sphygmology, acupuncture and moxibustion, Zhuyou (a witch doctor who treated ailments believed to be caused by witch craft), etc.

(1) Abundant in experience and practical in content

The two books are extremely abundant in content, summarizing the methods on diagnosis and treatment concerning internal medicine, surgical department, gynecology and pediatrics, as well as rich experience on acupuncture and moxibustion, medicinal knowledge, health preservation and dietary regimen. They also collect over 6,500 prescriptions before the Tang Dynasty, which come from the former famous physicians and the folk, as well as the minority groups and even foreigners. Many prescriptions in the two books become commonly used today, such as Rhinoceros Horn and Rehmannia Decoction for heat-clearing and blood-cooling, Spleen-Warming Decoction for yang-warming, purgation and dyspepsia-curing, Pubescent Angelica and Taxillus Decoction for qi-blood replenishing and wind-relieving, and so on, which make contributions to the development of formulas. Sun Simiao emphasizes comprehensive therapy in clinical practice, not only advocating the combination of acupuncture and medicine, but creating colored meridian-collateral diagram of human body. Moxibustion and massage are also commonly used in

疗法的积极倡导者，在书中专列"食治"一门，应用羊、鹿的甲状腺来治疗甲状腺肿，用动物肝脏治青光眼和夜盲，在防治营养缺乏性疾病方面取得了突出的成就，在世界医学史上也是重要创举。

his treatment. He also advocates food therapy and introduces some therapies in a volume, such as curing thyromegaly with thyroid of sheep or deer, treating glaucoma and nyctalopia with animal liver. It makes outstanding achievements in the prevention and treatment of deficiency disease and deserves to be a pioneering one in the medical history of the world.

（2）倡伤寒研究法

历代医家对《伤寒杂病论》的研究颇多，孙思邈对张仲景的学说研究有所发挥。他将《伤寒论》的内容较完整地收集在《千金翼方》中，为后世研究《伤寒论》提供了较可靠的版本。他所创立的从方、证、治三方面研究《伤寒论》的方法，成为后世以方类证的指南。

(2) Advocating the research method for febrile diseases

There are too many studies on *Treatise on Cold Damage and Miscellaneous Diseases* among doctors through the ages. Sun Simiao, however, further develops Zhang Zhongjing's theory and research. He includes the content of *Treatise on Cold Damage and Miscellaneous Diseases* completely in *Supplement to Essential Prescriptions Worth a Thousand Gold for Emergencies*, thus providing a reliable version of the book for further research. The research method he creates, analyzing the book from 3 perspectives (formulas, syndromes and treatment), becomes a guide for later generations to categorize syndromes by formulas.

（3）重视妇科和儿科疾病

孙思邈在临床研究中，非常重视妇科疾病和儿科疾病的诊治，他认为妇人和小儿是关系人类繁衍的大事，因此需要特别加以重视，并且在《千金要方》中将妇科疾病和儿科疾病辟为专卷，列于首位，详细论述妇、儿疾病诊治的特殊性和必要性，讨论了小儿护养的原则和方法，颇具科学性。这在当时以男性为主的封建社会中是极为难得的。

(3) Attaching importance to gynaecology and pediatric diseases

In the clinical research, Sun gives special attention to the diagnosis and treatment of women and children because he believes they are vital to human reproduction. So in the very beginning volumes of the book, he makes detailed statements on the specialty and necessity of the diagnosis and treatment of gynaecology and pediatric diseases and discusses scientific principles and methods of infant caring. It was quite advanced a thought in that male-dominated feudal society.

(4) 注重养生未病先防

孙思邈对于人体的养生也非常重视,他提出通过少思、少怒、少欲、摄精、养神、节食、熟食(食用熟的食物)、不偏食、运动等实现积极养生,强身长寿。这对于未病先防有很积极的意义。他在书中论述了很多积极的养生方法,如在日常劳作方面提出:"养生之道,常欲小劳,但莫大疲及强所不能堪";意思是人体保养自己,适度劳动有益身体,不可过度疲劳,超出身体负荷,否则会造成对身体的损伤;在饮食方面强调"安身之本必资于食",注意"食勿过饱"。他还总结了一套按摩养生法,使养生学成为有理论、有实践的学术,受到现代人的广泛重视。

(4) Laying emphasis on health preservation and disease prevention

Sun Simiao attaches great importance to life-cultivation, proposing that in order to keep body fit and strong, prevent diseases and reach longevity, men should worry less, annoy less, desire less, consolidate semen, nurture spirit, keep on diet, take prepared food, avoid dietary bias, and take physical exercises, and so on. What he advocates has positive meaning to disease prevention. Many positive life-cultivation methods are recorded in this book. For instance, in the aspect of daily work, the physical labour must be moderate and within an acceptable range, otherwise it will be harmful to health. In terms of diet, Sun argues that "To make the root of body safe, you must provide it with food" and "avoid overeating". He also summarizes a massage regimen, which makes regimen both theoretical and practical and gains wide attention from modern people.

(5) 强调地道药材

孙思邈本着"万物皆药"的思想,周游各大名山,实地采集和考察药物,努力发掘自然界中的药物价值,积累了丰富的药物学经验。他很注重地道药材,认识到药物的功效与产地有密切的关系,记载了当时133个州所产的地道药材519种。《千金翼方》中载录药物800余种,详述了药物的采集时节、加工炮制等,并对一些药物的药性进行了修正。

(5) Putting emphasis on authentic materia medica

Sun Simiao thinks all medicines are hidden in the nature, so he travels around famous mountains to collect and inspect various drugs, exploring their medical value and accumulating rich experience on pharmacology. He lays emphasis on authentic materia medica and recognizes close relationship between efficacy and place of origin. The book describes 519 kinds of drugs that could be found in counties (prefectures) at that time. In *Supplement to Essential Prescriptions Worth a Thousand Gold for Emergencies* more than 800 kinds of drugs are listed and expounded in detail with their proper harvesting, processing methods, etc. In addition, the properties of some drugs are also corrected in the book.

（6）论述医德医风

孙思邈在《备急千金要方》中写《大医习业》和《大医精诚》两篇，专门论述医德。他认为人的性命"贵于千金"，所以他的书就以"千金"而命名。他提出作为一名医生要注重个人的品德修养，做到"无欲无求"、"誓愿普救"；在对待病人态度方面要"普同一等"、"皆如至亲"；在个人的行为举止方面要端庄，"不得多语调笑……道说是非"，议论他人，也不可"炫耀声名"，不能因为偶然治好一个病人，就昂首仰面、自得自满的样子，认为自己天下无双，这是医生所应当避免的。孙思邈对医德的论述，可以说是最全面、最具体，这些基本医疗道德至今仍有着重要的现实意义。

(6) Discussion on medical ethics

There are two texts on medical ethics named "On the Absolute Sincerity of Great Physicians" and "On the Practice of Great Physicians" in the book *Essential Prescriptions Worth a Thousand Gold for Emergencies*. Sun thinks human lives are "worth more than one thousand gold", so the book is entitled with "thousand gold". He emphasizes that the superior doctors should cultivate personal virtues, "harbor no wishes and desires" and "commit himself firmly to the willingness to save every living creature". On the attitude to patients, a great doctor should "treat everyone fairly and act as if he were his close relative". In terms of personal behavior, "It is not permissible to be talkative and spread gossip to discuss other people." It is also inappropriate for someone who has accidentally healed a disease to "show off his reputation", to show conceit, and to announce that no one in the entire world could measure up to him. Sun Simiao's exposition on medical ethics is considered the most comprehensive and specific. These fundamental medical ethics still have important practical significance up to now.

三 学术价值

《千金方》作为中医史上的第一部医学百科全书，具有非常重要的影响，该书也代表了医学发展到唐朝时期的先进水平，这既是中医自身实践经验积累的成果，也是吸收外来文化、取各家之长的结果。此书不仅在国内影响极大，而且在亚洲国家传播广泛，在日本医学界，《千金方》被视为"人类之至宝"。作者孙思邈因对药物的深入研究和对药物学发展的突出贡献被后人尊为"药王"。

3 Academic value

As the first medical encyclopedia in the history of Chinese medicine, *Thousand Golden Prescriptions* has great influence and represents the advanced level of medical development in the Tang Dynasty. Its achievement is not only rooted in the long-term Chinese medicine practice, but also in the assimilation from the quintessence of foreign cultures and other doctors. It is widely spread in Asian countries and regarded as the most precious treasure of human beings in medical field of Japan. Sun Simiao is worshipped as "King of Medicine" for his outstanding contribution to the profound research of drugs and improvement of pharmacology.

12 刘涓子鬼遗方(Liu Juanzi Gui Yi Fang)

Liu Juanzi's Ghost-Bequeathed Prescriptions

一 书籍简介

《刘涓子鬼遗方》一书是目前我国所能见到的最早外科专书,书中记载了很多外科疾病,尤其对认识痈疽的病理特点、诊断鉴别方面均有非常详细的描述。该书传说是由晋朝的一位叫刘涓子的人在郊外巧遇"黄父鬼"时,"黄父鬼"遗留给他的,并因此而得书名。此书后来经刘涓子的后人传给北齐时期的龚庆宣,并经龚庆宣整理后而传世。原书又称为《痈疽方》。

1 A brief introduction to the book

Liu Juanzi's Ghost-Bequeathed Prescriptions (*Liu Juanzi Gui Yi Fang*) is the earliest extant monograph on surgery in China. It records a lot of surgical diseases, particularly detailed pathological characteristics and differential diagnosis of carbuncle. Legend had it that a man named Liu Juanzi in the Jin Dynasty encountered Huangfu Ghost in the suburbs, and the Ghost bequeathed this book to him, therefore the book was given this name. Later it was passed on to Gong Qingxuan in the Northern Qi Dynasty (550—577A. D.) and handed down to generations with Gong's arrangement. The original book was also known as *Prescriptions for Carbuncle*(*Yongju Fang*).

二 主要内容

原书为10卷,后来到宋朝时期的刻本为5卷。该书主要记述了金疮(刀枪外伤感染)、痈疽、疥癣等外科疾病,其中对痈疽的记载尤为详细。

2 The main content

The original book consists of 10 volumes. By the time of the Song Dynasty, there are 5 volumes in the block-printed edition. The book mainly gives an account of some surgical diseases such as metal-inflicted wound, carbuncle, scabies, among which carbuncle is particularly recorded in detail.

(1) 提出对痈疽早期的关注

书中指出了对于痈疽外科疾病,一般在初期常不引人注意,容易被忽视,故应在发病初期,尽早认识,了解此类外科疾

(1) Putting forward early attention to carbuncle

The book points out surgical diseases like carbuncle are likely to be ignored in the early stage. So at the onset, people should know as early as possible that these surgical diseases are characterized by quickly changing. Rapid

病的迅速变化特点,采取"急速治疗"的原则,不可拖延,否则就有可能使病情拖延和加重。

treatment should be adopted without any delay, otherwise the state of illness will be exacerbated.

(2) 提出痈疽的生长危险部位

书中提出长在嘴唇、鼻部周围以及耳旁的痈疽,尤应重视。这种观点和现代医学中注重鼻、唇附近颜面三角区及耳部周围炎症的观点是一致的,说明当时已经注意到这些部位是容易造成痈疽蔓延扩散的危险部位,如果疏忽会使病症扩散,引起全身感染,甚至可能危及生命。

(2) Proposing the dangerous location where carbuncle may occur in the body

The book mentions that the carbuncle near the lips, nose and ears should be taken seriously, which is in line with the viewpoint of modern medicine that inflammation of aural region and trigonum should be paid special attention to. This demonstrates that at that time the author has realized that these body parts are dangerous and easily suffered from the spread and diffusion of carbuncle. Negligence will result in the diffusion and general infection of the body, and even endanger the life.

(3) 提出痈疽的形成病机

书中针对痈疽的病机,指出是气血运行于血脉中,涩滞不畅,壅遏不行,进而蕴生火热,火热邪气腐肉为脓,从而形成痈。对于痈疽的诊断,书中介绍了非常实用有效的辨脓法,比如描述说:"痈大坚者,未有脓;半坚薄,半有脓;当上薄者,都有脓"。早在《伤寒杂病论》中就有关于痈肿的辨脓法,但主要是依据将手放在痈肿的部位,分辨皮肤的温度,热者为有脓,不热者为无脓。而《刘涓子鬼遗方》中的辨脓法则结合痈肿的坚硬度来判断是否已经形成脓,这种方法直至今天仍在临床沿用。

(3) Analyzing the pathogenesis of carbuncle

In regard to pathogenesis of carbuncle, the book points out it is caused by impaired qi-blood circulation. The stagnation and congealing of qi and blood in the vessels transform into to fire heat. If pathogenic heat continues to increase, it will lead to putridity and suppuration, eventually resulting in carbuncle. The book introduces practical recognition method of pus in the diagnosis of carbuncle. For instance, it records "if carbuncle is big and hard, there is no pus; if semi-hard, there is some; if the surface is thin, there is pus filled." In fact, the recognition method of pus had been mentioned as early as in *Treatise on Cold Damage and Miscellaneous Diseases* by touching the location where carbuncle occurs and feeling the temperature of the skin, that if it is hot, there is pus; if normal, no pus. However, the former method introduced in this book, recognizing carbuncle by its hardness, is still applied in clinical use to this day.

（4）提出内外兼治的原则

在治疗方面，书中讲究辨证施治，以局部病变的外治为主，同时又重视机体的内部调治。书中共记载有关内治、外治的处方140多首。外治的方法主要有针灸、使用外用药（如以黄连、大黄、水银等多种药物配成软膏、膏药治疗痈疽）、对痈肿的穿刺、切开、排脓引流等，引流的方法提出用火针穿刺排脓，既注意了消毒，又达到了排脓的目的。内治的方法则立足于清热解毒、活血化瘀和补气生津的原则，这三大原则不仅促进了以后外科病内治原则的形成，也成为后世外科"消、托、补"三法的确立基础。

(4) Putting forward the principle of combined internal and external treatment

Based on syndrome differentiation and treatment, the book puts forward the principle of combined internal and external treatment, in which, giving priority to external treatment of local lesions while attaching importance to internal recuperation. There are 140 prescriptions about internal and external treatment in the book. External treatment mainly covers methods as follows: acupuncture and moxibustion, taking drugs for external use e. g. combining several herbs like golden thread (huanglian), rhubarb and mercury into ointment and herbal paste, puncture, incision, evacuation and drainage of carbuncle, etc. As to drainage method, fire needling is proposed to puncture and evacuate pus, and at the time disinfection can be ensured. Internal treatment is based on three principles: heat-clearing and detoxifying, promoting blood circulation and removing blood stasis, tonifying qi and promoting the secretion of saliva or body fluid, which not only facilitate the establishment of internal treatment principle for surgical diseases, but also lay the foundation for the three methods of "*xiao*, *tuo*, *bu*" applied in surgical treatment of later generations. (*Xiao* method is applied to the carbuncle with no pus and can make it eliminate. *Tuo* method is used for middle period of the carbuncle while *Bu* method is for later period and aims at replenishing qi to promote tissue regeneration.)

三 学术价值

《刘涓子鬼遗方》作为我国现存最早的一部创伤外科专书，在继承前人基础上，又有新的进展，无论是预防、诊断、治则、方药等方面，都有某些独特见解。书中对于推动中医学的外科疾病治疗的专科化，无疑起到了积极作用。该书在外科学方面的成就具有一定的影响，历史上曾经被作为日本的医学教科书。

3 Academic value

As the earliest extant monograph on traumatology surgery, *Liu Juanzi's Ghost-Bequeathed Prescriptions* makes some new progress on the basis of inheriting the achievements by predecessors. It holds many unique insights in the aspects of prevention, diagnosis, therapeutic principle, formulas, etc. Undoubtedly, the book plays a positive role in promoting the specialization of surgical treatment in traditional Chinese medicine. The achievement the book has made in the field of surgery has broad implications and the book was once chosen to be the medical textbook in Japan.

13 仙授理伤续断秘方(Xianshou Lishang Xuduan Mifang)

Secret Methods of Treating Traumas and Fractures

一 书籍简介

中医学中的骨伤科形成较早,在中国最早的文字——甲骨文中,"疾"字是象形字,所呈现的就是表示人被矢镞射伤而需要治疗的图画。在我国较早的朝代——周朝时期(约相当于公元前1046—前256)就有"疡医",负责皮肤疾病的治疗,也负责处理"金疮"(刀枪所导致的外伤感染)、"折疡"(骨折以及发生感染的疾病)之类的骨伤科疾病。当时对不同程度的外伤已经有明确的界定,如:"皮曰伤,肉曰创,骨曰折,骨肉皆绝曰断"。到了汉代(约公元前206—公元220时期)在军队中已经设立有折伤簿,就是专门记录官兵折伤的医案。此后有关骨伤科的医学记载内容逐渐增多,如对创伤感染的认识,骨折、脱臼的复位固定,以及切开复位手术等,均有所创新。《仙授理伤续断秘方》约成书于唐朝的公元841—846年,是我国现存最早的一部骨伤科专著,作者是蔺

1 A brief introduction to the book

The science of orthopedics and traumatology was established in traditional Chinese medicine a long time ago. In the earliest Chinese characters (inscriptions on bones or tortoise shells), "疾" is a pictographic character demonstrating a picture on which a man is injured by arrowhead and needs medical treatment. In the relatively earlier Zhou Dynasty (1046—256B. C.), there were "surgeons" in charge of dealing with skin diseases, diseases of orthopedics and traumatology such as metal-inflicted wounds (wound infections caused by sword and spear) and bone trauma (fracture and infections). At that time, the different level of traumas had been clearly defined. For example, damage to the skin was called "abrasion"; injury on flesh was called wound; bone break was fracture; separation of bone and flesh was called break. In the Han Dynasty (206B. C. —220A. D.), there were already books of fracture which specially recorded medical cases of officials and soldiers. After that, medical records concerning orthopedics and traumatology gradually increased, such as cognition on trauma infections, restoration and fixation of dislocation and open reduction, which were innovative. The book, as the earliest extant monograph on orthopedics and traumatology, was written in the Tang Dynasty (around 841—846 A. D.). The author, Taoist Lin, was said to be a Taoist priest skilled in orthopedics. In his times, the government gave orders to

道人，据传是一位精于骨伤科的道士。在其生活的时代，由于政府要下令拆除寺庙，遣送僧道尼姑还俗从事生产劳动，他就到了江西的农村，将自己丰富的骨伤科理论知识和治疗技术，连同珍藏的骨伤科的专书《理伤续断方》，毫无保留地传授给一位经常帮助他耕耘的彭姓老人后就隐居起来，当地百姓因见他突然消失，便传说他是神仙下凡，将书更名为《仙授理伤续断秘方》。

remove temples, sending monks, nuns and Taoists to resume secular life and go in for productive labor, so he went to rural areas in Jiangxi province. He lived in seclusion after he passed on his abundant theoretical knowledge on orthopedics and traumatology, treatment techniques and precious monograph, *Methods of Treating Traumas and Fractures* (*Lishang Xuduan Fang*) unreservedly to an old peasant surnamed Peng who often helped him in farming. The local people spread words that he was an immortal descended to the earth because of his sudden disappearance. Then, the book was renamed *Secret Methods of Treating Traumas and Fractures* (*Xianshou Lishang Xuduan Mifang*).

二 主要内容

《仙授理伤续断秘方》一书记载了有关四肢骨折、脱位、颅骨骨折、腹部损伤、内伤、创伤后遗症等诸多疾病的诊断、治疗和方药。主要内容有：

2 The main content

The book records the diagnosis, healing and prescriptions of limb fracture, dislocation, skull fracture, abdominal injuries, internal injuries, trauma sequelae and so on. The main content is as follows:

(1) 系统地记述了骨折的治疗常规

书中记载了创伤骨折后的常规治疗方法和技术，包括创伤部位的局部冲洗、骨骼的牵引复位、创伤处的外治敷药、使用夹板固定骨折等多个步骤，为临床治疗提供了一套完整的治疗方案。书中还针对开放性骨折的处理，提出用快刀扩大创口，有利于减少创口感染发生，然后再清创、包扎。

(1) Systematic record of common practice of fracture treatment

The book records conventional treatment methods and techniques of bone fracture, including many procedures, such as wound irrigation, traction and reduction, wound dressings, fixation of splints, etc., which provides a complete therapeutical schedule for clinical treatment. Besides, in dealing with open fractures, the book also puts forward that "using sharp knife to enlarge the skin wound first so as to reduce wound infections, then cleaning the wound thoroughly and dressing the wound to help prevent infection".

（2）提出骨折复位固定的"动静结合"治则

针对骨折复位固定后的治疗，书中提出了"动静结合"的原则，即在保证骨折复位后有效固定的前提下，提倡患者伤肢的适当活动，以减少骨折痊愈后遗症的发生。这种固定与活动相结合的治疗原则给后世留下了重要影响，至今仍具有重要的临床价值和科学意义。

(2) Presenting the principle of "combination of being static and dynamic" for treating fracture reduction and fixation

In allusion to the follow-up treatment after fracture reduction and fixation, the book presents the principle of "combination of being static and dynamic", which means on the premise of effective fixation, proper functional exercises may help in reducing the occurrence of fracture sequelae. This principle exerts important impact on later generations and still has influential clinical value and scientific significance till now.

（3）发明了方便有效的治疗关节脱位方法

书中首次提出治疗肩关节脱位的"椅背复位法"，这种方法操作简便，容易实施，并且疗效确切。后来骨伤科的"架梯复位法"和至今在临床应用的复位法都是在这一原理基础上产生的。此外书中还介绍了关节脱位的常规诊断治疗方法，如"揣度"、"拔伸"、"捺正"，即医生用手切摸并诊断脱位的部位和程度、使用拔伸牵引和提按等手法将脱位的关节复位。

(3) Invention of convenient and effective treatment of dislocation

The method of "shoulder dislocation with chair back" is first invented in the book, which is not only easy and simple to handle, but also has definite curative effect. The later "resetting method with ladder" in orthopedics and traumatology and the resetting method in clinical application at present both are derived from the former one. In addition, the book also introduces common methods of diagnosis and treatment on joint dislocation. For example, the doctors touch the dislocation part, making diagnosis on the severity of dislocation, and then relocating the dislocated joints by applying some manipulations of pulling, traction, lifting and pressing.

三 学术价值

此书是一部既有文献价值、又能很好指导骨伤科临床实践的骨伤科专书。书中的理论学术思想起源于《内经》、《难经》的气血学说，并继承了《肘后救急方》、《备急千金要

3 Academic value

The book is a monograph on orthopedics and traumatology with both documentation and clinical value. The academic idea in the book originates from the theory of qi and blood in *Huangdi's Internal Classic* and *Classic of Difficult Issues*, inheriting the experience and achievements in orthopedics and traumatology in *The Handbook of Prescriptions for Emergencies*, *Important Prescriptions Worth a*

方》、《外台秘要》等有关骨伤科的经验成就，形成了以整复、固定、活动及内外用药为主体的治疗大法，初步奠定了骨伤科辨证、立法、处方与用药的基础，使辨证论治得以具体运用于骨伤科领域。书中所收载的外洗、外敷、内服等多种方药为后世骨伤科用药奠定了基础，也是中医骨伤科用药的典范，具有很高的临床应用价值。

Thousand Gold for Emergencies, *Arcane Essentials from the Imperial Library* (*Waitai Miyao*). The book develops therapeutical method which is centered on a set of procedures (reduction, fixation, activity, using drugs both internally and externally) and lays the foundation for differentiation, formation of treatment, prescription and pharmacy preliminarily, through which the syndrome differentiation and treatment can be actually applied in orthopedics and traumatology clinically. Many prescriptions collected and recorded in the book concerning external washing, external application and oral administration lay the foundation for prescribing in orthopedics and traumatology for later generations, setting a good example for medication in this field and holding great clinical value.

14 新修本草(Xinxiu Bencao)

Newly Revised Materia Medica

一 书籍简介

唐朝时期,社会经济有良好的发展,交通状况也较发达,在医学上药物的知识积累逐渐丰富,在实际临床中出现了许多新药和外来药,因此很有必要对药物做一次全面的整理和修订。公元657年,医学家苏敬根据这种状况向当时的政府提出了编修一部新的中药学专书的建议,经政府批准后下令由长孙无忌、李勣(jì)主持编修工作,由苏敬等20余人集体编写,并在全国范围内广泛收集道地药材,绘制药图,修订药物学内容,于公元659年撰成图文并茂、能充分反映当时药物发展水平的本草著作,书名《新修本草》(又称《唐本草》)。这部书是我国和世界第一部由国家编纂的药典,比欧洲著名的《纽伦堡药典》早800余年。

1 A brief introduction to the book

In the Tang Dynasty, the country witnessed a sound social and economic development as well as the traffic situation. With the gradually accumulated knowledge of medical drugs, it was necessary to make a comprehensive arrangement and revision of drugs as many new foreign drugs in clinical treatment had appeared. In 657 A. D., Su Jing, a medical physician, proposed compiling a new monograph on Chinese medicine to the government. After being approved, Zhangsun Wuji, Li Ji presided over the editing work while Su Jing and other 20 people were in charge of compiling. This book, *Newly Revised Materia Medica* (*Xinxiu Bencao*), also called *Materia Medica of Tang Dynasty* (*Tang Bencao*), was completed in 659 A. D. after extensively collecting samples of all medicinals from all over the country sketching medicine charts and revising pharmacology content, fully reflecting the level of drug development at that time. This book is the first pharmacopoeia in the whole world compiled by the State, over 800 years earlier than Europe's *Nuremberg Pharmacopoeia* (*Niulunbao Yaodian*).

二 主要内容

本书的编写遵循全面、实用和科学的态度精神,对前代的药物"详采博要"总结整理,对当时代的药物经验证后将

2 The main content

Guided by the comprehensive and practical principle and scientific attitude, the book gives a detailed summary of drugs from previous dynasties, collects all the drugs that being proved effective, revises former wrong records and

有疗效的药物修订编入书中，并修订以往内容有错的记载和补充新发现的药物和外来药物。全书共54卷，包括本草、药图、图经等三部分，其中本草20卷，药图25卷，图经7卷，目录2卷。本草部分记述药物的性味特点、产地、采制要点、治疗功效等；药图部分是根据药物实际形态描绘的图样；图经部分是对药图的文字说明。该书在内容上具有以下特点：

complements the newly discovered drugs and foreign drugs. The 54-volume book consists of three parts: herbal explanation, illustration and herbal description, of which 20 volumes are about herbal explanation, 25 volumes are illustrations, 7 volumes are description of illustrations, 2 volumes are contents. The part of "herbal explanation" describes the drug's properties, place of origin, collecting methods, potency, etc. Part of "illustration" provides paintings of the herbs while description is the textual explanation of medicinal herbs. The following will list the book's characteristics:

(1) 图文并茂的形式开创了药物学著作的新体裁先例

在编写过程中，政府发出"普颁天下，营求药物"的命令，从全国各地征集道地药材，并以药物的实物为标本，描绘药物图形，与文字相对照。因此书中"图经"部分，不仅用文字记载道地药材的产地、采药时日、形态鉴别以及加工炮制等内容，还专门列有药物的图，以作为识别药物的指导。这些绘图作为学习药物学知识、识别药物的重要依据是非常必要的。

(1) The form of illustration creating a new format on pharmacology books

In the process of compiling, the government issued an order of "informing the public, seeking for drugs", requiring to collect samples of all medicinals and then provide corresponding pictures of the samples and textual descriptions. Thus the section of "illustration" in the book not only records the origin of authentic medicines, harvesting time, morphological identification and processing methods, but also specifically lists pictures to identify herbs. These illustrations, as the important basis for learning pharmacology knowledge as well as the identification of herbs, are of great necessity.

(2) 体例清晰 一目了然

书中采用了统一清晰的体例，按照玉石、草、木、禽兽、虫鱼、果、菜、米谷及有名无用九类来分类，除有名无用的药物外，其他各类药物又分为上、中、下三品。每个药的正文用大号字体作单行行书，每个药的注文用小号字体，作双行书写。凡属于新增的药物都在最后标以"新附"二字，

(2) Clear arrangement with easy understanding

With a clear and unified style, the book classifies the herbs into 9 categories: jade, grass, wood, poultry and beast, insects and worms, fish, fruits, vegetables, rice and named unused drugs. In addition to named unused drugs, other drugs are divided into superior, common and inferior kinds. The text of each drug is written in single line and large font while the annotation part in double space and small font. The new drugs in the book are marked with "newly added" in the end. The annotation of drugs coming

凡药物的注解出自陶弘景的《本草经集注》一书的都在注解开头冠以"谨案"二字,这对了解古代药物资料的源流具有重要意义。

from *Collective Commentaries on Classics of Materia Medica* by Tao Hongjing all begins with the words "citation with prudence", which is of great significance in tracing the source of ancient drug-related materials.

(3) 补充了新增药物

本书在《本草经集注》730种药物的基础上,新增药物一百多种,共850种左右。所新增的一百多种药物大多很有价值,其中如蓖麻子、蒲公英等都是具有特效的药物,并且还收载了一些已为民间广泛应用的外来药物,如密陀僧、血竭、郁金、阿魏、刘寄奴、安息香、龙脑香、胡椒、薄荷、紫贝等。在食品方面记载了如鲫鱼、砂糖、油菜等的治疗作用,这些内容也是该书最早收载的。此外该书还介绍了一种叫银膏的制剂,即以白锡、银箔、水银调配而成,用于补牙。这种方法是世界上较早记载的补牙填充剂资料。

(3) Supplementing new drugs

Based on 730 kinds of drugs in *Collective Commentaries on Classics of Materia Medica*, this book adds more than one hundred kinds of new drugs, totaling up to 850 drugs. Most of which are of great value, such as drugs with special effect like castor bean, dandelion and so on. And it also reproduces some widely used civil foreign drugs, like litharge (mituoseng), dragon's blood (xuejie), turmeric root tuber (yujin), Chinese asafetida (awei), diverse wormwood herb (liujinu), benzoin (anxixiang), borneol (longnaoxiang), pepper fruit (hujiao), peppermint (bohe), Arabic cowry shell(zibei). In the food sector, it describes the therapeutic effect of carp, sugar and canola, which is also the earliest record. In addition, a quite earlier dental filler called silver paste is introduced , which is made by tin, mercury and silver foil.

三 学术价值

《新修本草》作为国内外最早的药典,普查了全国药物,总结了历代药物学文献,由国家颁布,内容丰富,叙述准确,所以一经问世就广泛流传。此书不仅成为医生的必读之书,而且亦成为医生与药商用药、售药的法律依据。邻国朝鲜、日本等对此书也非常重视,公元10世纪日本曾下令医学界"凡医生皆读苏敬《新修本草》",反映出该书在国内外医学界的重要地位。

3 Academic value

As the earliest pharmacopoeia in the world promulgated by the state, the book covers the national drugs and sums up all the ancient pharmaceutical literature. It is rich in content and accurate in description, so it was spread widely once published. This book not only became a must-read for doctors, but also became a legal basis for treatment and drug sale between doctors and drug providers. Neighboring countries like Korea and Japan also attached great importance to this book. In the 10th century, Japan had ordered "all the doctors must read *Newly Revised Materia Medica* by Su Jing", which reflected the important status of the book in the medical field of home and abroad.

15 食疗本草(Shiliao Bencao)

Materia Medica for Dietotherapy

一 书籍简介

中医学很早就有关于食物治疗疾病的描述，人们在日常生活中也会运用食物去调养身体。《食疗本草》是我国现存最早的古代营养学和食物治疗专著。该书为唐代孟诜(shēn)所撰写，孟诜(约公元621年—713年)是唐朝医学家，从小喜好医学，善于学习，掌握了不少医药知识，尤其对于食物所具有的治疗效果非常了解。他所撰写的《食疗本草》详细地记载了很多食物的治病效果，是中医学对食物性味功效的补充和整理。

1 A brief introduction to the book

There were descriptions about treating diseases by dietary therapy in Chinese medicine a long time ago. People built up the health by taking food in their daily life. *Materia Medica for Dietotherapy* (*Shiliao Bencao*) is the earliest extant monograph on ancient nutriology and dietary therapy. It was compiled by Meng Shen (621—713A. D.), a medical scientist in the Tang Dynasty, who was a good learner and was fond of Chinese medicine, therefore he had a good grasp of relevant knowledge, especially the therapeutic effect of food. The book gives a detailed record of curative effect of various foods, supplementing and rearranging foods' nature, flavor and efficacy in Chinese medicine.

二 主要内容

《食疗本草》全书共分三卷，收集药物二百余种，对其食性、功能、主治都做了详细的辨析和论述，并鉴别食物之间的异同，指出食物服用的禁忌事项，对食物的外部形态、产地等也都有描述。另外对南北不同地域的饮食习惯、孕妇和产妇以及小儿的饮食宜忌等方面也作有记述。书中所记载的食物多为人们日常所用的，如谷物、蔬菜、果品、肉类和动物脏器等。书中记

2 The main content

Materia Medica for Dietotherapy consists of 3 volumes in total and keeps a record of over 200 drugs. It makes the discrimination and discussion on drugs' nature, functions, and efficacy, identifying the similarities and differences among foods, emphasizing the counterindications, describing their external morphology and places of origin. Besides, it also introduces different eating habits between southern and northern regions, healthy food and food taboos for the pregnant, women and children. Most foods recorded in the book are from the daily diet, such as grain, vegetables, fruits, meat, animals' visceral organs, etc. Lots of descriptions

载了很多食物的治病作用，如用绿豆有助于通行十二经脉；大豆捣涂后可以治疗一切皮肤的毒肿和治疗男女的阴部肿大等；茄子可以用醋调后敷在皮肤的肿胀处，以清热解毒；用茄子的根可以煮汤后浸泡脚部，治疗脚部有冻疮的人；鲤鱼用白水煮食可以治疗身体的水肿，帮助气血下行通畅等等；大枣、醋、酒等具有解毒的作用。

on foods' therapeutic effects are included in the book. For example, mung bean contributes to blood circulation through twelve meridians; mashed soybeans can be used to treat all skin swelling and tumidness in humans' private parts. Stirred with vinegar, eggplants can be applied upon tumid parts to clear away heat and toxin; boiled root of eggplant in foot bath is curative to chilblain. Eating carp boiled with water can eliminate body edema and help to promote downward circulation; Chinese date, vinegar and spirit serve the function of detoxication.

三 学术价值

《食疗本草》原书已佚失，其内容可见于《证类本草》、《医心方》等书中。该书汇集了唐朝以前对食物的医疗运用经验，补充了食物的药用价值，内容丰富，至今对指导人们使用食物治疗疾病仍具有较高的研究价值。

3 Academic value

The original version of *Materia Medica for Dietotherapy* has been lost and its content can be seen in *Classified Materia Medica* and *The Essence of Medicine and Therapeutic Methods* (*Yi Xin Fang*) (Japanese name: *Ishimpo*), and so on. The book is rich in content, aggregating medical experience of dietotherapy before the Tang Dynasty and replenishing the medical value of foods, which still holds great value of research in guiding people to apply dietotherapy for disease treatment.

16 本草拾遗(Bencao Shiyi)

Supplement to Materia Medica

一 书籍简介

《本草拾遗》一书是对《新修本草》的补充,作者是唐朝的药学家陈藏器(约公元687—757年),自小就随父辈采集药物,辨识百草,长大后研习各类本草医书,认为《新修本草》虽然对中药做了汇总整理,但是也还有遗漏的内容,因此就于公元739年撰写了《本草拾遗》10卷(今已经佚失)。虽然该书已佚失,难以查考所记载的药物总数,但宋朝的《证类本草》一书引该书药物488种,明朝的药学家李时珍所著的《本草纲目》引该书药物368种,比引用的《新修本草》114种多3倍余。书中所载的药物,有许多是不被前人所记录收载的,大大增加了中药的药物数量。

1 A brief introduction to the book

Supplement to Materia Medica (*Bencao Shiyi*) is the complement of *Newly Revised Materia Medica*, which was written by Chen Cangqi in the Tang Dynasty (approximately 687—757 A. D.). The author had gathered herbs with his father at an early age so he could identify hundreds of herbs. After growing up, he studied all kinds of medical books on material medica. He considered that although *Newly Revised Materia Medica* made a gathering and arrangement of medicinal herbs, there were still omissions. Therefore, he wrote *Supplement to Materia Medica* (10 volumes in all) in 739 A. D., which no longer exists now, so the sum of medicines it records are not possible to examine. However, *Classified Materia Medica* in the Song Dynasty quoted 488 medicines from the book; *Compendium of Materia Medica* (*Bencao Gangmu*) by Li Shizhen in the Ming Dynasty quoted 368 medicines from the book, the number of quotation was over 3 times more than that of *Newly Revised Materia Medica* (114 medicines). Many of the recorded medicines in the book were never included before, which expanded the number of Chinese medicines greatly.

二 主要内容

《本草拾遗》书中的内容包括3部分,其中序例1卷,相当于药物总论;拾遗6卷,详细地描述了许多药物的药名、产地、性状、采制、性味、毒性、药

2 The main content

There are 3 parts in the book: one exordium (pandect of medicines), 6 volumes of gleanings (description on drug names, place of origin, shapes and properties, collection and processing, nature and flavor, toxicity, efficacy, indications, prohibitions) and 3 volumes of commentary

效、主治和禁忌等；解说3卷，主要是考证品种，订正讹误，辨析形态与性味相似易于混淆者。书中内容丰富广博，对于中医药学贡献放大。

(mainly examination of varieties, correction of errors, differentiation of similar forms, properties and flavors of drugs). The book is rich in content, making great contributions to TCM.

（1）新增药物和扩充药物功效和用法

(1) Supplement of drugs and expansion of drug efficacy and application

《本草拾遗》增补了许多药物，仅矿物类就增加了110多种。所补充的药物来源广泛，既有来自内陆的，又有来自沿海地区的；既有汉族又有少数民族的药物，还包括国外传入的药物。对许多药物的临床应用方法都有所发展，如指出葛根经水磨而澄取的淀粉可以入药，味甘性寒，其生津止渴的效力较传统的葛根为优。后世沿用了对葛根粉的使用方法，临床多用作清热除烦。书中还记载了热敷物理疗法，如用夏季河中的干热砂让患者伏坐其中以治疗风湿关节疼痛、功能受限等病，这种沙浴疗法直至现代在民间也还有不少人在应用；还有使用化学方法治疗外科疾患的描述，如用草蒿烧为灰洒上水后可治疗身体皮肤的息肉病症，这恐怕是将无机碱的腐蚀作用应用于治疗息肉的较早案例。

A lot of drugs are supplemented in *Supplement to Materia Medica*, including at least 110 kinds of mineral drugs. They come from various sources, including inland or coastal areas, Han and minority nationalities, and overseas. The clinical application methods of many drugs are further developed. For example, it points out the powder that are extracted from grinding kudzuvine root (gegen) tastes sweet, cold-natured and can be used as medicine. Its efficacy of helping produce saliva and quench thirsty is much better than traditional kudzuvine root. The later generations inherit the application of kudzuvine root powder to clear heat and relieve fidget clinically. There are also content on physical therapy of hot compress, for example, patients who have rheumatoid arthralgia and functional limitations could sit among hot dry sand from the river in summer. This sand bath therapy is still applied among many people at present. There are also descriptions of treatment of surgical diseases by chemical methods. For instance, incinerated artemisia annua mixed with water can cure polyposis, which is probably an early case that utilizes the corrosive effect of inorganic base to treat polyp.

（2）创造了药物和药剂的分类法

(2) Establishment of the classification method of drugs and formulas

书中将中药的药物性能归纳为10类：宣、通、补、泄、轻、重、滑、涩、燥、湿，起初作

The book reduces the properties of herbal drugs into ten categories: dispelling, obstruction-removing, tonifying, purgative, light, heavy, lubricant, astringent, drying and

为临诊处方基本法则，后发展成后世的"十剂"方剂分类法，至今仍为中医界应用。这种分类法为后世方剂学按功能分类奠定了基础。

moistening. The ten-category classification method, as a basic law of clinical diagnosis, has still been used so far in traditional Chinese medicine, which lays the foundation for classification of formulas according to efficacy in later ages.

(3) 纠正以前部分药物学知识的讹误

作者对于之前的药物学著作指出了一些存在错误之处的记载，如指出"接骨木"这一味实际有小毒，《新修本草》中记载无毒是错误的；姜黄性热不冷，而《新修本草》则记载为性寒；他还指出前人将菊科属植物泽兰与兰草相混的错误等。

(3) Correction of some previous errors in pharmocological knowledge

The author points out some errors in the previous works on Chinese materia medica. For example, elderberry is actually slightly toxic, so the record of being non-toxic in *Newly Revised Materia Medica* is not right; Turmeric (jianghuang) is hot in nature while in *Newly Revised Materia Medica* it is described as cold-natured. The confusion of predecessors between hirsute shiny bugleweed herb (zelan) which belongs to the composite family and bluegrass (lancao) is also stated.

三 学术价值

《本草拾遗》收罗广博，且大部分记载是正确的，既吸收了众多的民间医学成就，也勇于实践，无论是理论还是临床应用都有自己的创见。明朝的药学家李时珍评此书"博极群书，精核物类，订绳谬误，搜罗幽隐，自本草以来，一人而已。"《本草拾遗》是继《新修本草》之后唐朝贡献最大的民间药物学专著，所收药品中不少被后世药学著作引录为正品，另外日本医籍《医心方》等均有引用，证明域外医家对此书也非常重视。

3 Academic value

Among its wide collections, most content in *Supplement to Materia Medica* is correct. The book absorbs various achievements in folks and takes bold medical practice, putting forth innovative ideas both in theory and clinic. The pharmacologist Li Shizhen of the Ming Dynasty remarks, "*Supplement to Materia Medica* is counted as the best work on materia medica which absorbs the content of a variety of books, classifies herbs precisely, corrects mistakes of previous medical books, gleans hidden information". It is a monograph on materia medica which makes the greatest contribution in the Tang Dynasty after *Newly Revised Materia Medica*. Many herbs that are included in *Supplement to Materia Medica* are cited as certified medication items by pharmaceutical works in later generations. In addition, some content in it is quoted by *The Essence of Medicine and Therapeutic Methods* , a Japanese medical work, which proves that foreign medical experts also attach great importance to the book.

17 外台秘要(Waitai Miyao)

Arcane Essentials from the Imperial Library

一 书籍简介

《外台秘要》是唐朝及唐以前的医学文献辑录而成的综合性医书。作者是王焘,曾担任国家官员,后主要负责管理国家图书,并能够有条件广泛地阅览各种文献资料。因为母亲生病他学习医学,并随从一些名医研究医术,且能够有机会接触到一些罕见的医书,因此作者就把大量的医学文献统一整编,于公元752年撰写成方药和理论结合的综合性著作《外台秘要》,使前人的理论研究与治疗方药全面系统地结合起来。

1 A brief introduction to the book

Arcane Essentials from the Imperial Library is an integrated medical book compiled from medical literature in the Tang Dynasty and before. The author Wang Tao, who had been served as a national official and was mainly in charge of national library later, had the chance to read large amount of documents. As his mother was ill, he followed some famous doctors to learn medical skills. Having access to some rare medical books, Wang Tao reorganized amounts of medical literature and completed the comprehensive book *Arcane Essentials from the Imperial Library* in 752 A. D., making theoretical research and clinical prescriptions made by predecessors integrated comprehensively.

二 主要内容

《外台秘要》共包括40卷,全书分1 104门(目前核实为1048门),载方6 000余首,其中1—20卷记载内科疾病,21—22卷记载五官科疾病,23—24卷记载瘿瘤、瘰疬、痈疽等病,25—27卷记载二阴病,28—30卷记载金疮、恶疾等疾病,31—32卷记载丸散等成方,33—34卷记载妇人病,35—36卷记载小儿

2 The main content

The book consists of 40 volumes with 1,104 categories and more than 6,000 formulas. Among which, respectively, internal medical diseases, ENT diseases and goiter and tumor, scrofula and carbuncle are registered in volumes 1 to 20, 21 to 22 and 23 to 24. Diseases of anterior and posterior orifices, metal-inflicted wound, foul diseases and patent prescriptions like pills and powder are covered in volumes 25 to 27, 28 to 30 and 31 to 32 respectively. Diseases of women, children and that induced by galalith intake are included in volumes 33 to 34, 35 to 36 and 37 to 38 separately. And moxibustion therapy, insect or animal

病,37—38卷记载服食乳石而导致的疾病,39卷记载灸法,40卷记载兽伤及畜疾。每门记述都先理论阐述后记载药方,其中理论部分主要以巢元方的《诸病源候论》为主,方药部分则选自《千金方》者最多。其余所选各书,均注明有书名卷次,使后人能借此得以了解晋唐期间许多已经散佚的方书内容。该书的特点包括:

bites and diseases of livestock are discussed in volumes 39 and 40. The account of every category falls into narration of theory in the first and the record of formulas afterwards. The former part is mainly about the *Treatise on Causes and Manifestations of Various Diseases* by Chao Yuanfang while the latter part mostly from *Thousand Golden Prescriptions*. Other selected books are marked with the titles and volume number, so the later generations could see formulas that is lost during the Jin and Tang dynasties (265—907 A. D.). The book can be characterized as follows:

(1) 较全面地整理和保存了大量的古代医学文献

《外台秘要》全书搜罗详备、笼而不杂、先论后方、次序井然。书中引证的方书共69种,集医方近万首。所引资料均注明书名和卷次,以便于查核,为医学文献的整理创立了范例,并保存了如《小品方》、《崔氏方》等不少今已亡佚的方书内容。

(1) Comprehensively arranging and storing the ancient medical documents

Arcane Essentials from the Imperial Library is rich in content, systematic and orderly in structure. 69 medical books on formulas are quoted in it, integrating near 10,000 formulas. The titles and volume numbers of the cited documents are marked out for the convenience of checking, creating a paradigm for organizing medical documents and preserving much content of medical books that have been lost nowadays such as *Classical Prescriptions* (*Xiaopin Fang*) and *Prescriptions of Cui Family* (*Cuishi Fang*).

(2) 内容广泛

书中内容包括了内、外、骨、妇、儿、传染病、皮肤、五官、畜病等所有医科的诊治,搜集、整理并推广了大量的民间单验方。如"许明疗人久咳欲死方"、"苍梧道人陈元膏"等,并对这些方药详细地记载了其疗效、治疗范围和来源。

(2) Wide-ranging content

The book covers diagnosis and treatment of many departments, including internal medicine, surgery, orthopedics, gynecology, paediatrics, infectious diseases, dermatology, ENT and animal diseases. A lot of proved recipes from the folk are collected, organized and popularized such as "prescription for treating chronic cough by Xu Ming" and "Chenyuan Paste (Cangwu Daoren Chenyuan Gao)", whose curative effect, indications and the sources are also recorded in detail.

(3) 肯定了大批有效的方药

书中对很多中药临床上的特异疗效作了肯定的描述。如常山、蜀漆(常山苗)可以治疗疟疾;用动物肝脏可以治疗夜盲症,并且已经不单限于羊肝一种,牛肝、猪肝等亦被采用;治疗颈瘿(甲状腺肿大)用海藻、昆布等。书中所载的"石膏汤"、"黄连解毒汤"、"葱白七味饮"等许多方剂千余年来被有效地应用着。

(3) Affirming highly of effective prescriptions in large amounts

The book affirmly describes specifically the curative effects of some Chinese medicines in clinic, for instance, malaria can be cured by antifebrile dichroa root (changshan) and sprout of antifebrile dichroa root (shuqi); hesperanopia can be treated by animal livers, which include lamb liver, beef liver and pork liver, etc. And herbs such as seaweed and kelp can be used for the treatment of goiter. Many formulas registered on the book, like "Gypsum Decoction (Shigao Tang)", "Coptis Detoxification Decoction (Huanglian Jiedu Tang)", and "Scallion Decoction with Seven Ingredients (Congbai Qiwei Yin)", are effectively applied in clinic for more than one thousand years.

(4) 对疾病认识和治疗有新的发展

书中较突出地对伤寒、肺结核、疟疾、天花、霍乱等传染病做了描述,如具体记载了肺结核盗汗、午后潮热、面部潮红以及日益消瘦的症状;描述了天花发疹、起浆、化脓、结浆的全部过程且对预后判断做了明确的说明;书中所记述的"消渴者……每发即小便至甜",即对糖尿病的尿糖异常的诊断方法比西方同样的认识早近900多年;书中很系统地记述了治疗白内障的"金针拔障术",记述了"一针之后,豁若开云而见白日"之功效;书中首次记载了用白帛浸染法检验小便颜色的方法来鉴别诊断黄疸病的轻重及病情变化,并可据此观察对黄疸的治疗效果。此外书中还汇集了唐以前的多种治疗方法,如

(4) Making new development of disease recognition and treatment

The book focuses on the description of some infectious diseases, such as typhoid, tuberculosis, malaria, smallpox, cholera, etc. Tuberculosis is characterized by night sweats, afternoon tidal fever, congested cheeks and emaciation. Definite narration is given about the whole course of smallpox, including eruption, plasma, fester and its prognosis. The description of "the sweet-tasting urine of patients with diabetes..." in the book infers that the diagnostic method based on the abnormal glucose in urine appears 900 years earlier than western countries. "Couching Techniques for Cataract" is introduced systematically, with vivid description of "just like the sun appears as the clouds disperse after needling". It is the earliest record that using dipped white cloth to check the color of urination can diagnose and observe the curative effect of the condition of yellow jaundice and change of disease. Additionally, a number of treatments before the Tang Dynasty are accumulated in the book, such as moxibustion, fumigation

灸、薰吸、吹、蒸以及多种切实可行的急救法如儿科食道异物治疗等。

and inhalation, blowing and steaming, as well as many available first aids such as treatment on the pediatric foreign-body in the esophagus.

三 学术价值

《外台秘要》是唐朝一部总结性医学著作，曾被赞为“世宝”，整理者王焘因此被誉为文献整理的“大师”。从医学文献整理角度看，《外台秘要》保存了不少佚失的古医籍内容，具有很高的文献价值。对此清代医家徐灵胎曾赞许说：“历代之方，于焉大备……唐以前之方，赖此书以存，其功亦不可泯。”唐朝以后的医学教育也将《外台秘要》选作教科书，认为“不观《外台》方，不读《千金》论，则医人所见不广，用药不神”。该书也传播到了邻国朝鲜和日本，书中大量的内容被引用，如朝鲜的《医方类聚》和日本的《医心方》中都大量引用该书资料，由此可见此书在医学界的重要地位。

3 Academic value

Arcane Essentials from the Imperial Library, a summary work of medicine in the Tang Dynasty, had been praised as "world treasure". Wang Tao, therefore, was honored as "a great master" of organizing documents. From the perspective of medical documents arrangement, the book is of high documentary value for it preserves a large amount of ancient medical works that have been lost. So that's why physician Xu Lingtai in the Qing Dynasty had commended that "The book records numerous prescriptions of past dynasties, and thanks to the book, the prescriptions before the Tang Dynasty are preserved". It was also recognized as a textbook for medical education after the Tang Dynasty. It was believed that "physicians are short of much insight and accurate medication without reading *Arcane Essentials from the Imperial Library* and *Thousand Golden Prescriptions*". Furthermore, the book was transmitted to Korea and Japan, a lot of information of it were cited in *Collection of Medical Prescriptions* (*Yifang Leiju*) from Korea and *The Essence of Medicine and Therapeutic Methods* from Japan, which fully proved the importance of the book in the medical world.

18 经效产宝(Jingxiao Chanbao)

Valuable Experience in Obstetrics

一 书籍简介

《经效产宝》是我国现存较早的妇产科专书，对后世医家有着广泛而深入的影响，具有很高的文献学和临床学价值。可惜曾经一度流失，现今所见已非原书，乃3卷辑佚本。作者是唐朝的名医昝(zǎn)殷，临床方面擅长妇产科，且精通医理，于公元852年将前人有关经、带、胎、产及产后诸症的经验效方及自己临床验方撰著成书。

1 A brief introduction to the book

Valuable Experience in Obstetrics (*Jingxiao Chanbao*) is the earlier Chinese monograph on gynecology and obstetrics, which has extensive and profound influence on later physicians with a high philological and clinical value. Unfortunately, because it had once been lost, what can be seen today is not the original book—three volumes through compilation of scattered documents. The author was the celebrated doctor Zan Yin in the Tang Dynasty, who specialized in obstetrics and gynecology in clinic, and was proficient in principles of medicine. In 852 A. D., he completed the book by combining efficacious prescriptions related with menstruation, leukorrhea, pregnancy, delivery and postpartum syndromes with his own clinical prescriptions.

二 主要内容

《经效产宝》一书共分三卷，52篇，378方。其中上卷为经闭、带下及妊娠各方，中卷为坐月、难产内容，下卷为产后各种病症等。全书论述较简明扼要。

2 The main content

Valuable Experience in Obstetrics consists of three volumes with 52 articles and 378 formulas and discusses the content in a concise way, among which, the first volume describes amenorrhea, vaginal discharge and pregnancy, the second volume tells of puerperium care and dystocia, the third one discusses all kinds of postpartum syndromes.

（1）详细描述了妊娠反应

作者临床经验丰富，观察详细，记载了妇女妊娠反应的

(1) Detailed description of the pregnancy reaction

The author has rich clinical experience. With careful observation, he describes the women's pregnancy reaction to the point and in detail, such as feeling upset, dizzy and

表现"心中愦愦(头昏的样子),头旋目眩,四肢沉重,懈怠,恶闻食气,好吃酸咸果实,多卧少起,三月四月多呕逆,肢节不得自举者",描述详尽而且扼要。其中所附3首处方,用人参、厚朴、白术、茯苓之类药物健脾利水,橘皮、生姜、竹茹等化痰止呕,对于妊娠反应的疗效较为可靠。对于孕妇在妊娠期提出以养胎保胎为要,治疗上重视调理气血、补益脾肾。

nauseous, heavy in limbs, slack, or prefer sour and salt flavor fruits, lying more than walking; or frequent vomiting for 3-or 4-month pregnancy, the incapability of lifting limbs. There are three prescriptions attached to this book, of which, drugs like ginseng (renshen), officinal magnolia bark (houpo), white atractylodes rhizome (baizhu) and Indian bread (fuling) can be used for spleen invigoration and water drainage; drugs like orange peel, fresh ginger (shengjiang) and bamboo shavings (zhuru) for phlegm resolution and vomiting relief. These drugs are all effective for pregnancy reaction. For pregnant women, the book gives priority to nourishing the fetus and preventing miscarriages. In treatment, it pays attention to regulating the qi and blood and replenishing the spleen and kidney.

(2)对先兆流产和难产的认识

对胎动不安(先兆流产)的病理提出两种观点,一是"因母病而动胎",一是"胎不坚(即胎儿先天发育不良)"而导致,这与现代医学的认识相类似。其所拟用的安胎方用续断、艾叶、当归、干地黄、阿胶等类药物,有补肾、滋阴和安胎的良好作用。书中还重点讨论了难产,如对难产之一的"胎衣不下",作者认为与"产时用力过度",或粗暴地牵引脐带等原因有关,与现代医学认识也相近。对难产妇人主张"内宜用药,外宜用法",即用滋补强壮的药物给产妇内服以增强体力,再加上外治手术助产使胎儿娩出,其原则至今也有指导意义。

(2) The recognition on threatened miscarriages and dystocia

The book presents two views about the pathology of fetal irritability (threatened abortion), one is "because of the mother's disease", the other is because "fetus is not strong (i. e., fetus is inborn dysplasia)", which are similar to the understanding of modern medicine. The prescription for preventing abortion contains himalayan teasel root (xuduan), argy wormwood leaf (aiye), Chinese angelica, dried rehmannia root (gandihuang), donkey hide gelatin (ejiao) and other drugs which have functions to tonify kidney and nourish yin and tocolysis as well. The book also focuses on dystocia, such as "placenta retention". The author considers it is related to "excessive force during delivery" or violently pulling the umbilical cord, which is also similar with modern medical knowledge. The woman who is difficult in giving birth should be treated "with the principle of combined medications and manipulations", namely, using tonic drugs to enhance strength combined with external midwifery surgery to deliver the infants, which is still instructive nowadays.

(3) 对产后病认识丰富

书中对"产后烦渴"、"产后乳结成痈"及"产后热结便秘"等产后病的病因和所用方药作了记载,如"产后烦渴"是因产时"水血俱下"伤津所致;产后乳痈是因"产后不曾乳儿,亦结成痈";"产后热结便秘"不主张内服攻下药,而采用外用药物通大便,审慎而有效。尤其对产后血晕的急救,指出"须速投方药,若不急疗,即危其命也",并可用烧红的秤砣淬醋熏蒸,作为产后血晕的应急措施,实用而简便易行。

(3) Full understanding of postpartum diseases

The book records some pathogeny and prescriptions about "postpartum polydipsia", "postpartum mastitis" as well as "postpartum constipation". For example, "postpartum polydipsia" is caused by fluid damage due to "sinking of both blood and water" and "postpartum mastitis" is due to "never breastfeeding". As to "postpartum constipation", topical drugs are proposed to relax the bowels rather than taking offensive purgative, which are prudent and effective. For the first-aid of postpartum anemic fainting, it points out that "taking herbs instantly, or it will be life-threatening". What's more, fumigating and steaming method with red-hot iron mound quenched with vinegar can be used as the emergency measure for this syndrome, which is easy, practical and convenient.

三 学术价值

《经效产宝》围绕妊娠、分娩、产后等病症详论证治,保留了唐以前产科方面的经验方药,为后世妇产科之法则,对中医妇产科学的发展有一定贡献。

3 Academic value

Valuable Experience in Obstetrics discusses the syndromes and treatment in detail about pregnancy, delivery, and postpartum symptoms, retaining the previous empirical prescriptions about obstetrics before the Tang Dynasty, being set as a law of gynaecology and obstetrics for future generations. It makes a contribution to the development of Chinese medicine in obstetrics and gynecology.

19 太平圣惠方(Taiping Shenghui Fang)

Taiping Holy Prescriptions for Universal Relief

一 书籍简介

《太平圣惠方》是宋朝的政府诏令所编修的一部大型医药方书,由翰林医官王怀隐等人负责,广泛收集宋朝以前的方药书籍及当时的民间验方,检验并分门别类整理医药验方,历经14年时间,集体编著而成。《太平圣惠方》成书于公元992年,并由政府下令刻印并出版,发行于全国,让各地设立专门负责人员保管该书。该书内容丰富,所记载方药涉及临床各科,所搜集的医方,较能反映当时代的医学水平,具有很高的临床实用价值。

1 A brief introduction to the book

Taiping Holy Prescriptions for Universal Relief (*Taiping Shenghui Fang*) is a large-scale medical formulary compiled by Wang Huaiyin, the head of the Imperial Academy of Medicine, together with other officials of the department under the command of the Song Dynasty government. They spent 14 years widely collecting, examining and classifying prescription books before the Song Dynasty and the folk remedies of the time. The book was completed in 992 A. D. and then mint-marked and published across the country under the government order. Moreover, in adherence to government order, every local authority appointed a functionary in charge specially to take care of the book. The book is rich in content, covering prescriptions in various clinical departments. The collection of medical prescriptions in the book is a relatively good reflection of the medical level at the time and holds high value in clinical practice.

二 主要内容

全书共包括100卷,分脉法、处方用药、五脏病症、外科、骨伤、胎产、妇、儿、丹药、食治、补益、针灸等1 670门,收录方药16 834首。书中强调医生治病必须辨阴阳、虚实、寒热和表里,务使方随证

2 The main content

The book consists of 100 volumes with 1,670 categories and 16,834 prescriptions, covering sphygmology, prescriptions, syndrome of five zang-organs, surgery, bone fracture, pregnancy and delivery, gynecology, pediatrics, pellets, diet therapy, tonifying, acupuncture and moxibustion and so on. It emphasizes the importance of differentiation between yin and yang, deficiency and excess, chills and fever, exterior and interior, so as to compose the formula according to syndrome differentiation and to take medicines

设，药随方施，并论述了病因病机、证候与方剂药物的关系。

according to composed formula. In addition, the relationship among etiology, pathogenesis, syndrome and prescription is also discussed in the book.

该书的体例是按照脏腑和各科病症分类，先理论阐述后记载方药。在每一种门类的病症下，都是先引用《诸病源候论》一书中的理论为总论，然后再汇集方药，体现了理、法、方、药较完整的辨证论治体系。书中选用的药物，不但品种多，而且有些是前代罕用或不用的。此外书中很多记载都是目前现存最早的记录，如关于外科“五善七恶”的说法，外科“内消”与“托里”的治疗原则，小儿急惊风和慢惊风的分辨，眼科白内障使用“金针拔障术”的详细过程等，此外还首次确立了妇科的经、带、胎、产的编排序例，成为后世所依循的标准。

The book is classified by zang-fu viscera and syndromes of different departments, introducing the theory first and then followed by prescriptions. When talking about each category, it begins with quoting the theory from *Treatise on Causes and Manifestations of Various Diseases* as pandect and then collects and lists prescriptions concerned, which presenting the complete system of syndrome differentiation and treatment on the basis of theory, method, prescription and medicine. Medicines collected in the book are not only abundant in kind but also include drugs that are rarely used or never used in previous dynasties. Besides, there are many earliest extant records, such as, “five good symptoms and seven bad symptoms”, therapeutic principles of internal dissolution and replenishing qi in surgical department, the discrimination of acute infantile convulsions and chronic infantile convulsions of children, detailed process of cataract extraction surgery used by golden needle. In addition, the arrangement sequence of menstruation, morbid leucorrhea, pregnancy and delivery is also established for the first time, which becomes the standard followed by later generations.

三 学术价值

《太平圣惠方》因为记载内容极其丰富，被后人认为内多有“异域瑰奇”之品；在经络、俞穴以及刺灸、治法等方面，也都有所发挥提高。该书卷帙庞大，保存了两汉迄于隋唐间的许多名方，同时也保存了许多已散佚的医书内容，因此在医学界具有相当大的影响。

3 Academic value

On account of its rich content, *Taiping Holy Prescriptions for Universal Relief* is considered to be a magnificent and rare work to some extent. It makes some development on meridians and collaterals, acupoints, acupuncture and moxibustion and therapy, etc. The book is of great influence in medical field because it preserves not only many well-known prescriptions from the Western Han and Eastern Han dynasties to the Sui and Tang dynasties but also numerous content from medical books that had been lost.

20 本草图经(Bencao Tujing)

Illustrations on Materia Medica

一 书籍简介

《本草图经》是我国医药学历史上第一部由政府编绘而成的药物图谱,又名《图经本草》。该书的编写是由宋朝的政府组织,下诏从全国各地征集药物标本及药图,并命令注明开花结实、采收季节和功用,对于进口的药物则询问收税机关和商人,辨清来源,选出样品,送交政府。这种全国性的药物大普查,不仅成为世界药学史上的壮举,也为编写《本草图经》奠定了基础。该书于公元1058年由官员苏颂(公元1020—1101年)主持编撰,在公元1061年完成。书中所绘制的药物图谱力求形象逼真,所描述的文字力求准确精当;凡不能分辨的药物,则兼收并存。

1 A brief introduction to the book

Illustrations on Materia Medica (*Bencao Tujing*), also known as *Tu Jing Ben Cao* , is the earliest documented Chinese government-compiled pharmacopoeia in the history of medicine. It was organized by the government of the Song Dynasty, who ordered to collect and provide drug specimens and graphs throughout the country, marking out the blossom and bearing, harvesting seasons and functions. As for imported medications, it was commanded to inquire tax keepers and businessmen for their sources, so that the samples could be selected and delivered to the government. The general survey of drugs nationwide not only became a world feat in the history of pharmacology, but also laid the foundation for the compiling the book. It was mainly compiled and edited by officer Su Song (1020—1101A. D.) in 1058—1061A. D. The drug graphs drawn in the book were strived to be vivid, while the words to be accurate. All undistinguished drugs were also kept in the book.

二 主要内容

《本草图经》共有21卷,其中包括目录1卷。书中载药780种,其中新增民间草药103种,并在635种药名下绘制药图933幅。书中对

2 The main content

Illustrations on Materia Medica consists of 21 volumes, including one volume of catalogue. 780 kinds of drugs are registered in the book, among which, 103 folk herbs are newly added, and 933 pictures totally cover 635 kinds of drugs. The book focuses on the discussion of the origin and

药物的来源和鉴别也做了重点讨论，把辨药和用药结合起来，并收载有大量单方验方，还特别强调药物产地，对每种药物的不同产地详加考证和比较，提出质量最好的为道地药材。因此《本草图经》的实用性很强，深为后世医家所赞颂。

identification of drugs, combining the differentiation of drugs with medication. A number of folk or single-drug prescriptions and classical prescriptions are recorded. Particularly, it emphasizes where the drugs are produced. The different origins of each drug are compared and researched in detail, and then the medicine with top-quality are recommended as genuine regional materia medica. Above all, the high practicability of the book is eulogized by the physicians in later generations.

此书引用宋朝以前的文献200多种，集历代药物学著作和中国药物普查之大成，记载了多种药用植物和药用动物或其副产品，以及大量重要的化学物质，记述了食盐、钢铁、水银、白银、汞化合物、铝化合物等多种物质的制备。对不同地方的地理自然状况、历史发展和经济发展等方面也有记述。

The book cites more than 200 kinds of documents written before the Song Dynasty, epitomizing all pharmacology classics in the past dynasties and medicine survey in China, recording a variety of medicinal plants, animals and their by-products, as well as a great quantity of crucial chemical substances. Besides, the preparation of many materials are described in it, such as salt, steel, mercury, silver, mercury compound, and aluminum compound, etc. The geographical situation, historical development and economic growth are also narrated.

三 学术价值

《本草图经》是一部历史上承前启后的药物学巨著，书中继承了祖国多年来的古代医药学遗产，补充了自己的研究心得和发现，绘制了大量的药物图形，加以文字说明，准确地记载了各种药物的产地、形态、性质、用途、采集季节、炼制方法、鉴别方法与配伍、禁忌等，图文并茂，使用准确方便。原书虽然早已散佚，但其主要内容则保留在《证类本草》和《本草纲目》两部书籍中。《本草纲目》的作者李时

3 Academic value

Illustrations on Materia Medica is a great pharmacopoeia inheriting the past and breaking new ground for the future, preserving ancient medical legacy for thousands of years, supplementing research note and discovery, drawing a large number of illustrations with accurate text descriptions, including origin, appearance, characteristics, usage, collection, processing, identification, compatibility and contraindication, etc. Though the original text of the book had been lost for a long time, its main contents were documented in two later publications: *Classified Materia Medica* and *Compendium of Materia Medica*. The author of the latter, Li Shizhen, a famous pharmacologist in the Ming

珍是明朝的著名药物学家，他对《本草图经》的科学价值予以很高评价，认为"考证详明，颇有发挥"，并在其著作中引用《本草图经》多达74处，开创了明朝集大成的药物学巨著《本草纲目》之先河。

Dynasty, spoke highly of the scientific value of the book, holding that "textual research is well proved and greatly developed as well". In his book, *Illustrations on Materia Medica* had been cited as many as 74 times, which created the precedent for the later great work on materia medica—*Compendium of Materia Medica* in the Ming Dynasty.

21 证类本草(Zhenglei Bencao)

Classified Materia Medica

一 书籍简介

《经史证类备急本草》简称《证类本草》,是宋朝时期重要的药物总结性书籍,由出身世医之家的名医唐慎微(约公元1056—1093年)编撰而成。唐慎微学习刻苦,举止朴实,具有高超的医术,医德高尚,长期在民间行医,治病不分贵贱贫富,不避风雨寒暑,有求必应。在临床治疗过程中,他常常不取报酬,只求供给良药验方。因此人们都愿意与他接近,把所知道的好方良药告诉他,即使从书籍中发现的医药记载也都"必录以告",这些都为唐慎微积累广博知识和丰富经验创造了有利条件。该书约成于公元1082年,是在广泛收集民间和历代文献有关药物的记载基础上编撰而成,是宋朝最著名的药物学著作。

1 A brief introduction to the book

Classified Materia Medica from Historical Classics for Emergency, short for *Classified Materia Medica*, was an important summative book on materia medica in the Song Dynasty. It was compiled by Tang Shenwei (about 1056—1093A. D.), a prominent doctor born in a family that had been practicing traditional Chinese medicine for generations, who was diligent in learning and unpretentious in demeanor. With superb medical skills and noble medical ethics, he practiced medicine among the people for a long time, giving patients immediate treatment no matter they were rich or poor and what the weather was like. Since he always asked for no remuneration but just providing effective and proved medicines, people were willing to approach him and told him effective prescriptions that they knew, even including the record discovered from books. All of these had created favorable conditions for Tang Shenwei to accumulate wide knowledge and rich experience. The book, accomplished in about 1082 A. D., was complied on the basis of broad records accumulated from folk and past documents on materia medica. It was the most famous work on materia medica in the Song Dynasty.

二 主要内容

全书内容非常丰富,共32卷,载药1 558种,其中476种是以往药物书籍未曾记载的,

2 The main content

The book is rich in content with 32 volumes in total and 1,558 drugs. Among which, 476 drugs are not recorded previously, such as cinnabar artificial (lingsha) and

如灵砂、桑牛等皆为首次载入。每味药均附有药图可供查阅时参考；在药物性味、主治、鉴别以及归经理论等方面均详加阐述和考证；书中还提供了丰富的药物炮制内容，在每味药之下附以制法，既收录了《雷公炮炙论》中300种药物的炮制方法，又收载了《本草经集注》中的有关法则，为后世提供了宝贵的药物炮制资料，也在药物炮制文献资料的保存方面有重要贡献。

书中附方共3 000余首，有关方药的理论有1 000余条，对方剂学也有很大的贡献；在药物有效成分的提炼方面，书中记载了“秋石”（尿甾体性激素）阳炼及阴炼两种制备法，其中阳炼法成功地应用了皂甙沉淀甾体这一特异反应，属于世界上提炼“性激素”的最早记载。

mulberry longicorn (sangniu). There is a detailed exposition and research on the properties and flavors, indications, identification and meridian tropism theory of drugs in this book and an illustration attached to each drug for reference. What's more, it provides plentiful information about drug processing and the specific processing methods. The processing methods of 300 drugs in *Master Lei's Discourse on Medicine Processing* and some relevant rules in *Collective Commentaries on Classics of Materia Medica* are all collected and recorded in this book, not only providing valuable materials of drug processing for later generations, but also making a significant contribution to the preservation of these documents.

In addition, more than 3,000 formulas and over 1,000 related theories included in the book also make great contributions to Chinese medical formulas. In the aspect of drug extraction of the active constituents, the book records two processing methods of urinary steroid hormones—yang extraction (urinary extracted through dissolving, filtering, evaporating, drying, sublimating and crystallizing) and yin extraction (natural extraction), of which the yang extraction method successfully utilizes the specific reaction that saponin precipitates steroid. This is the earliest record of "sex hormone" extraction around the world.

三 学术价值

《证类本草》成书印刷后受到普遍的重视，后来政府在此书的基础上先后多次增补，作为国家药典颁行，流传后世并成为药物学著作的范本。特别值得一提的是该书摘录古代文献十分慎重，以采录原文为主，翔实完整记录原著，从而保留了许多古籍的原始面貌。

3 Academic value

Classified Materia Medica received widespread attention after its publication. Afterwards, the government made supplements for several times based on the original book and enacted it as a national pharmacopoeia. So it was passed down over generations and served as the model for medicinal works. The meticulous attitude towards excerpt from ancient literature was particularly worth mentioning. It gave first place to the excerpt of original articles, keeping accurate and complete account of original books, and thus the original appearance of many ancient works has been preserved.

书中选辑书目达二百余种,除医药著作外,还包括"经史外传"、"佛书道藏"等,使后人在古代文献大量散佚的情况下,仍可借此了解有关原文,具有很高的文献学价值。明代著名药学家李时珍撰写《本草纲目》时,以此书作为蓝本,并高度评价该书说:"使诸家本草及各药单方,垂之千古,不致沦没者,皆其功也。"

There are up to over 200 selected articles in the book. Except for medical parts, it also covers other subjects, such as "classics, histories and unofficial biographies" and "Buddhist and Taoism scriptures" etc., making the later generations still able to access the related original articles under the condition that numerous ancient documents are lost. So it is of great literature value. Li Shizhen, a famous pharmacist in the Ming Dynasty, just took this book as the original script when he was writing *Compendium of Materia Medica*. He spoke highly of the book, "Thanks to *Classified Materia Medica*, various herbs and prescriptions of many schools are preserved and handed down to generations."

22 小儿药证直诀(Xiaoer Yaozheng Zhijue)

Key to Medicines and Patterns of Children's Diseases

一 书籍简介

《小儿药证直诀》又名《小儿药证真诀》、《钱氏小儿药证直诀》,是中国儿科医学的奠基之作,是我国现存最早的儿科专著,在儿科发展史上占有重要地位。在宋朝时期儿科已成为独立的专科,当时著名的儿科医学家钱乙(公元1035—1117年)从事临床研究40余年,积累了丰富的临床经验。史料记载他曾因诊治皇族孩子有功被授予翰林学士。钱乙逝世后不久,其弟子阎孝忠将他的理论和经验整理成书,于公元1119年编辑成《小儿药证直诀》一书。本书是中国早期内容比较完整并载有病案的儿科重要专著。

1 A brief introduction to the book

Key to Medicines and Patterns of Children's Diseases (*Xiaoer Yaozheng Zhijue*), also named *Qian's Key to Medicines and Patterns of Children's Diseases*, is the foundation of Chinese pediatrics and the earliest monograph on pediatrics extant in China, occupying an important position in the history of pediatrics. In the Song Dynasty, pediatrics had already been an independent speciality. Qian Yi (1035—1117A. D.), a prominent pediatrician at that time, had been engaged in clinical research for over 40 years and accumulated rich clinical experience. According to history records, he was once awarded as a member of the Imperial Academy due to his meritorious treatment for royal kids. Shortly after his death, his disciple Yan Xiaozhong sorted out and compiled his theories and experience into the book *Key to Medicines and Patterns of Children's Diseases* in 1119 A. D., which was a significant and relatively complete work on pediatrics with records of medical cases in early China.

二 主要内容

全书共分为3卷,卷首附有《钱乙传》一篇,其中上卷是脉证治法内容,主要讨论小儿的生理、病理、五脏辨病论治等,列举常见小儿病症80余条;中卷详细地记载了经钱乙治疗的小儿危重疑难病案23

2 The main content

The book consists of three volumes along with a biography of Qian Yi in the preface. Volume One is about the therapeutic methods of pulse syndromes, mainly discussing physiology, pathology, syndrome differentiation and treatment of five zang-organs and listing more than 80 common syndromes of pediatric disease. Volume Two records 23 intractable and critical cases dealt by Qian Yi in

个，充分展示了他的医学观点；下卷诸方主要介绍了钱乙的临床经验方122首，论述了儿科方剂的配伍和用法。

detail, fully demonstrating his medical viewpoints. Volume Three mainly introduces 122 empirical formulas applied by Qian Yi in clinic, expounding compatibility and usage of pediatric prescriptions.

（1）在儿科诊疗方面提出了很多新理论

《小儿药证直诀》在儿科的诊疗方面颇有创见，对后世儿科的理论与实践具有重要的指导作用。该书在理论上系统地论述了小儿的生理、病理特点，认为小儿生理上属于"五脏六腑，成而未全，全而未壮"的状态；病理上则"易虚易实"、"易寒易热"；在诊断上要全面观察，包括如面部、眼目、指爪等多个部位，并注重通过观察小儿面部和眼部的神色来诊察和区别五脏状态，发展了小儿望诊；在治疗上提出要以"柔润"为原则，反对"痛击"、"大下"和"蛮补"，必须审慎用药。在小儿护理方面也有一定的认识，指出治疗同时要调理，以善其后。总之，该书在儿科疾病的诊断治疗方面形成了一套以幼儿五脏为纲的辨证施治体系。

(1) Putting forward many new theories in the pediatric diagnosis and treatment

Key to Medicines and Patterns of Children's Diseases puts forward some original ideas in the pediatric diagnosis and treatment, providing theoretical and clinical guidance for later generations on pediatrics. The book expounds on the characteristics of physiology and pathology in theory systematically. It holds that, in physiology, children's internal organs are not fully developed; in pathology, they are vulnerable to the manifestation of deficiency or excess, cold or heat; in diagnosis, overall observation is required, including many body parts like face, eyes, and fingers. It thus develops pediatric inspection by examining and differentiating the condition of five zang-organs after observing their faces and eyes. In treatment, it advocates the principle of being moderate and using medicines with caution instead of over-dosing or taking excessive tonic. Meanwhile, the book also has its own ideas on pediatric nursing, pointing out that treatment should be combined with regulation so as to recuperate well. In short, taking five zang-organs differentiation as the guiding principle, the book has formed a set of system in the pediatric diagnosis and treatment.

（2）创制了很多儿科实用有效的方剂

根据以上理论，钱乙创制了一些儿科专用方剂，如治疗痘疹初起的升麻葛根汤，治疗小儿心热的导赤散，治疗小儿脾胃虚弱、消化不良的异功

(2) Creating lots of practical and effective pediatric prescriptions

According to the theories above, Qian Yi creates some prescriptions specialized for pediatrics, such as Decoction of Rhizoma Cimicifugae and Radix Pueraiae (Shengma Gegen Tang) to treat pox at the onset stage, Redness-Removing Powder (Daochi San) to treat fire and heat syndrome of the heart meridian, Extraordinary Merit Powder (Yigong San)

散，以及治疗小儿肾阴不足的六味地黄丸等，皆有较好的疗效。这些补泻五脏的儿科方剂为后世医家所常用，也成为后世医家临症化裁的重要依据。对于痘疹(天花)、水痘、麻疹等发疹性儿科传染病也有丰富的治疗经验，并能进一步鉴别，详细记载了这些疾病的表现、诊断和治疗方法。

to treat spleen-stomach deficiency syndrome and indigestion, Six-Ingredient Rehmannia Pill(Liuwei Dihuang Wan) to treat syndrome of kidney-yin deficiency. With good efficacy, all these pediatric prescriptions for reinforcement and reduction of the five zang-organs are often used by later physicians and become an important basis for them to determine the diagnosis and treatment in clinic. As for eruptive infectious diseases in the pediatrics, such as smallpox, chicken pox and measles, Qian Yi also accumulates rich treating experience, and he can further identify these diseases, whose manifestations, diagnosis and treating methods are all recorded in detail.

三 学术价值

《小儿药证直诀》是儿科学形成独立体系的标志，对中医儿科学的发展做出了重要的贡献。钱乙本人也被誉为“幼科冠绝一代”、“儿科鼻祖”。钱乙继承和发展了《内经》和历代诸家学说，“概括古今，又多自得”，他首先把五脏辨证的方法运用到儿科临床，针对五脏虚实，立补泻主治的诸方。

钱乙的学术思想对后世的影响远远超过了儿科范畴，已遍及内、外、妇各科。“五脏辨证”方法对后世著名医家张元素的脏腑标本寒热虚实用药很有启迪。钱乙根据古方“金匮肾气丸”化裁制成的“六味地黄丸”不仅成为中医滋阴补肾的代表方，而且为后世很多名方的出现奠定了基础。

3 Academic value

Key to Medicines and Patterns of Children's Diseases marks the formation of independent system of pediatrics. It makes great contributions to the development of TCM pediatrics. Qian Yi himself is also honored as “the most outstanding pediatrician of his generation” and “pediatric originator”. He inherits and develops *Internal Classic* and medical thoughts of different schools in the past dynasties, “Achieving more than what others have concluded since ancient times”. It is Qian Yi who first applies syndrome differentiation of five zang-organs into pediatric clinic, making reinforcing or reducing prescriptions according to different syndromes of the five zang-organs.

The impact of Qian's academic thoughts on later generations is far beyond the field of pediatrics, covering many departments such as internal medicine, surgery, and gynecology. The method “syndrome differentiation of five zang-organs” serves as an enlightenment to Zhang Yuansu, a famous physician in the later generation, who often administers drugs according to different syndromes of zang-fu organs marked by cold, heat, deficiency and excess. Six-Ingredient Rehmannia Pill, which is modified by Qian Yi on the basis of ancient formula Golden Cabinet Kidney-qi (Jingui Shenqi Wan Pill), not only becomes the TCM representative formula of nourishing yin and tonifying kidney, but also lays the foundation for the emergence of many famous prescriptions in later ages.

23 太平惠民和剂局方(Taiping Huimin Hejiju Fang)

Formulary of the Bureau of Taiping People's Welfare Pharmacy

一 书籍简介

宋朝时期政府负责药材的买卖,并设立了专门买卖药材的机构,制造、出售丸散膏丹和药酒。当时把制剂药物的机构称为"和剂局"。《太平惠民和剂局方》是我国医学史上第一部由国家颁行的成药专书和配方手册,又名《和剂局方》,由宋朝的太医局编写而成。该书起初是太医局的成药处方配书,后曾多次增补修订刊行,而书名、卷次也有多次调整,于公元1151年经校订后改名为《太平惠民和剂局方》,成为目前流传的版本,是官方药局的制剂规范。

1 A brief introduction to the book

In the Song Dynasty, the government was in charge of the management and business of medicinal herbs. A specialized agency, which was called "The Pharmacy Bureau", was set up to manufacture and sell pills, powder, plaster, pellet and medicinal liquor. *Formulary of the Bureau of Taiping People's Welfare Pharmacy* (*Taiping Huimin Hejiju Fang*), is the first monograph on patent medicine and formula manual issued by the government in the history of medicine. It was compiled by Bureau of Imperial Physicians in the Song Dynasty. In the beginning, the book was the bound volume of patent medicine formulas. In 1151 A. D., it was renamed *Formulary of the Bureau of Taiping People's Welfare Pharmacy* after being supplemented, revised and published for many times later and became the popular version and preparation criterion for official pharmacy.

二 主要内容

《太平惠民和剂局方》共10卷,附指南总论3卷,分伤风、伤寒、一切气、痰饮、诸虚、痼冷、积热、泻痢、眼目疾、咽喉口齿、杂病、疮肿、伤折、妇人诸疾及小儿诸疾共14门,载方788首。

2 The main content

The book has 10 volumes, including 3 volumes attached as pandect. It is classified into 14 categories with 788 formulas in total, covering common cold, cold damage, all diseases related to qi, phlegm retention, all deficiency, obstinate cold syndrome, accumulated heat, diarrhea, eye disease, diseases of mouth, teeth and throat, miscellaneous diseases, sores, traumatic fracture, and diseases of women and children.

（1）丰富的方剂内容

所收方剂均是民间常用的有效中药方剂，每个方剂后都详细列出适用的病症、方剂的药物组成和用量，此外还详细地说明了药物的炮制、保存等内容。书中所记载的方剂及其剂型都来源于实践，而且有相当一部分是继承前人的宝贵经验，具有很高的临床价值，其中如至宝丹、牛黄清心丸、苏合香丸、紫雪丹等药物是高热神昏或中风昏厥等危急病症的必用药；黑锡丹、活络丹、藿香正气散、失笑散、香连丸等都是临床公认疗效卓著的常用药。妇科常用的四物汤、逍遥散，儿科常用的肥儿丸等药物也均出自此书。

（1） Rich content of prescription

The formulas in the book are all effective and commonly-used among the people. Their indications, composition and dosage, as well as processing and storage are all listed and explained in detail. Formulas and dosage forms registered in the book are all rooted in practice, and a large amount of them are precious experience inherited from former generations, which has great clinical value. For example, medicines like Supreme Treasured Pill, Bovine Bezoar Heart-Cleaning Pill, Styrax Pill and Purple Snowy Powder are required for emergency such as syncope due to high fever and stroke; some medicines are commonly used and universally recognized as the highly effective in clinic, such as Black Tin Pill, Collaterals-Activating Pill, Patchouli Qi-Righting Powder, Powder for Dissipating Blood Stasis and Aucklandia and Coptis Pill, etc. Other medicines such as Four Ingredients Decoction and Peripatetic Powder often used in the department of gynecology, as well as Chubby Child Pill used in the pediatrics all originate from this book.

（2）丰富的成药剂型制备方法

《太平惠民和剂局方》中的方剂大多数都是成药。该书介绍了非常丰富的成药剂型，所列出的剂型有十余种之多，如丸、散、膏、丹、锭、饼、香等；书中研究了许多成药的制备方法，记叙了185种中药饮片的炮制标准，还详细地描述了如水飞、醋焠、纸煨、煅、浸、煎、蒸、炒、火焙等炮制方法；发展了用酒、醋炮制药物的方法，如酒炒、酒蒸及醋炒药物，酒制可以助活血，醋制可以增强收敛，说明炮制目的已不单纯是抑制药物的毒性作用，而是进一步

（2） Plentiful preparation methods of dosage form

Formulas in the book are mostly patent medicines. It introduces plentiful dosage forms and lists more than ten of them such as pill, powder, plaster, pellet, troche, cake, aroma, etc. Many preparation methods are studied and processing standards of 185 kinds of herbal medicines are narrated. Also, the processing methods are described in detail, such as grinding with water, quenching with vinegar, roasting with paper, calcining, soaking, decocting, steaming, stir-frying, fire baking, etc. The book also develops processing methods with spirit and vinegar, for instance, stir-frying with spirit, steaming with spirit and stir-frying with vinegar. Processing with spirit can invigorate blood circulation while processing with vinegar can enhance astringency, which indicates that processing not only aims to inhibit toxicity of medicines but also further enhance or improve their efficacy.

增强或改进药物功效。

此外在丸药加工技术上也有新发展，增加了糊丸、水泛丸和化学丸剂等，发展了朱砂衣、青黛衣、麝香衣等多种丸衣。书中还提出了多种服药方法，如温酒送服、米饮送服、煎去渣服等内服法以及贴、涂、点眼、搐鼻、吹喉等外用法。

In addition, there is new development on pill-processing technology, for example, newly added forms such as flour and water paste pill, water pill and chemical pill, many new parcels of pills made of cinnabar, natural indigo and musk. Lots of new methods of taking drugs are suggested, including methods for oral administration such as taking with warm spirit, rice soup and taking without dregs, as well as methods for external application like pasting, applying, eye-dripping, nasal-applying, and larynx-blowing.

三 学术价值

《太平惠民和剂局方》是一部流传较广、影响较大的临床方书。这部书对成药的发展和推广做出了重大贡献，书中许多方剂至今仍广泛用于临床，特别是很多方剂立法完善，组方缜密，代表了中医方剂学的成就。该书被认为是"官府守之以立法，医门传之以为业，病者传之以立命，世人习之以成俗"的重要书籍，足见《太平惠民和剂局方》对医学影响是何等广泛和巨大。

3 Academic value

Formulary of the Bureau of Taiping People's Welfare Pharmacy is a clinical monograph on formulas with widespread influence, making great contribution to the development and popularization of patent medicine. So far, a lot of formulas in the book are still widely applied clinically, some of which, especially, with well-established therapeutic methods and rigorous-formed formulas, represent the achievement of formulas of Chinese medicine. This book is remarked as an important book " for governments to preserve to legislate, for physicians to impart to practice medicine, for patients to share to survive and for people to accustom themselves to this custom", which is sufficient to show how wide and great influence it makes on medicine.

24 三因极一病证方论(Sanyin Jiyi Bingzheng Fanglun)

Treatise on the Three Categories of Pathogenic Factors and Prescriptions

一 书籍简介

中医学对病因的认识源于《内经》,奠基于《金匮要略》,至宋朝时期发展形成病因学说,成为整个中医理论体系的一个组成部分。这一时期的病因学说代表作为陈言撰写于公元1174年的《三因极一病证方论》,简称《三因方》。作者陈言认为"医事之要,无出三因","倘识三因,病无余蕴",并在前人对病因认识基础之上,将病因分为三类,即内因、外因、不内外因。

1 A brief introduction to the book

Stemmed from *Internal Classic* and based on *Synopsis of Prescriptions of the Golden Chamber*, the understanding of disease cause in traditional Chinese medicine (TCM) developed into etiology theory in the Song Dynasty, which became a part of TCM theoretical system. The representative work of etiology in this period was *Treatise on the Three Categories of Pathogenic Factors and Prescriptions* (*Sanyin Jiyi Bingzheng Fanglun*) composed by Chen Yan in 1174 A.D., which was called in simplified name as *Formulas for Three Etiologies* (*Sanyin Fang*). The author thought that the most important issues in medical practice were nothing else than three categories of causes. The illness could be clearly known as long as the cause could be determined. On the basis of the predecessors' understanding of etiology, he divided the causes of disease into three categories—internal, external, and neither internal nor external.

二 主要内容

《三因极一病证方论》共有18卷,卷1至卷2前半部为医学总论,卷2后半部至卷18分别叙述内、外、妇、儿各科病症,并附有治疗方剂,共分180门,载方1 500余首。书中方药与理论结合颇切实用,其中有相当一部分

2 The main content

The book consists of 18 volumes. Volume 1 to the first half of volume 2 are the general overview of medicine. The second half of volume 2 to volume 18 discuss various syndromes of different departments including internal medicine, surgery, gynecology, pediatrics and their corresponding prescriptions for treatment. This part is divided into 180 classes and registers more than 1,500 prescriptions. The combination of prescriptions and theories in the book is quite practical, among which a portion of

方剂未记载于宋朝之前的医学文献。

prescriptions have not been registered in medical literature before the Song Dynasty.

(1) 提出三因学说

(1) Putting forward the theory of three etiologies

在病因研究方面,作者在张仲景的"三因致病说"基础上进一步阐发,将病因分为三类:一为外因,如外界的风、寒、暑、湿、燥、热六淫之气和瘟疫之气,认为外因"先自经络流入,内合于脏腑";二为内因,如人的喜、怒、忧、思、悲、恐、惊七情,认为"七情,人之常性,动之则先自脏腑郁发,外形于肢体,为内所因";三为不内外因,如生活不节、饮食饥饱、虎狼毒虫、虫兽所伤、金疮折跌、畏压缢溺等。书中所列的病症也以三因为依据而分门别类。

On the basis of Zhang Zhongjing's theory of "Three Pathogenic Factors", the author further classifies pathogenic factors into three categories. The first category is external cause, such as six climatic and pestilent pathogens of wind, cold, summer heat, dampness, dryness and fire. He holds that external pathogens invade the human body via meridians and collaterals first, and then converge in the viscera. The second category is internal cause, such as seven emotions (joy, anger, worry, overthinking, sorrow, fear and fright). As normal emotions of human body, seven emotions are first triggered from the viscera and then manifested outwards on the body. The third category is neither internal nor external cause, such as immoderate life, improper diet, poisonous insects, injuries by insect or animal, traumatic injuries, overstrain, hanging and drowning. Syndromes listed in the book are also classified according to the three categories of etiology.

(2) 三因学说在临床的应用

(2) Clinical application of the theory of three etiologies

这三种致病的病因既可单独致病又能相兼为病,彼此并非完全割裂,因此在临床上的辨证论治要审察证候而求其病因,并指出病因对于辨证治疗的作用"凡治病,须识因,不知其因,病源无目"、"不知其因,施治错谬,医之大患,不可不知",强调在治疗上也要审明三因,"治之之法,当先审其三因,三因既明,则所施无不切中"。

The three etiologies are not completely split to each other in that they may lead to diseases separately or jointly. Therefore, clinical syndrome differentiation and treatment mainly focus on determining the disease cause by observing the syndromes. The book points out the effect of disease cause on syndrome differentiation and treatment, holding that the doctor must make causes clear before treatment. Giving treatment without knowing the etiology is the biggest problem in medical practice. Only by observing the etiologies and making them clear can all the therapies be effective.

三 学术价值

《三因极一病证方论》全书条理分明，辨析严谨，文字简要，有证有论，有法有方。书中将三因学说作为论述的重点，使中医病因学说更加系统化、理论化。三因分类的原则一直被后世研究病因的医家所遵循，对研究中医病因学说和各科临床辨证论治等均有参考价值。

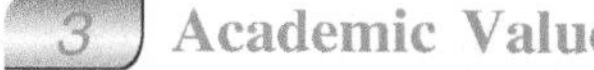

3 Academic Value

With sufficient arguments and methods of diagnosis and treatment, *Treatise on the Three Categories of Pathogenic Factors and Prescriptions* is coherent, rigorous and concise. The discussion on the theory of three etiologies is given priority in the book, making the etiology of Chinese medicine more systematic and theoretical. The theory of three etiologies has always been followed by physicians who study etiology in later generations and it has reference value on the research of etiology in TCM and clinical syndrome differentiation and treatment as well.

25 妇人大全良方(Furen Daquan Liangfang)

A Complete Collection of Effective Prescriptions for Women

一 书籍简介

宋朝时期的妇产科学发展比较突出,出现了一批妇产科的专著,其中最有影响的代表作是陈自明的《妇人大全良方》。作者陈自明出身于三代医家,精于妇产科学的研究,认为妇科病最为难治,尤其产科的各种病症常常容易有生命危险。他博览历代医家的著述,汲取诸家之长,并继承家传的良方和验方,于1237年撰写成《妇人大全良方》。该书又名《妇人良方大全》、《妇人良方集要》、《妇人良方》等,是一部内容系统而丰富的妇产科专书,长期为后世所应用。

1 A brief introduction to the book

In the Song Dynasty, obstetrics and gynecology developed rapidly and a batch of monographs on obstetrics and gynecology emerged, among which, the most influential masterpiece was *A Complete Collection of Effective Prescriptions for Women* (*Furen Daquan Liangfang*) written by Chen Ziming, whose family had practiced medicine for three generations. He was specialized in studying obstetrics and gynecology, considering that gynecopathy was the most difficult disease to deal with, especially its different symptoms were likely to be fatal. He read widely about writings from doctors through the ages, learned from their merits, and inherited the effective prescriptions handed down in the family. The book was compiled in 1237, which was also named *Collection of Effective Prescriptions for Women*. Since it was a specialized book on obstetrics and gynecology with rich and systematic content, it has been applied by the later generations for a long time.

二 主要内容

《妇人大全良方》共有24卷,分为8种门类,包括调经、众疾、求嗣、胎教、候胎(诊断)、妊娠、产难(即难产)和产后,共260多篇论述。书中在每论之下都加有按语,并大多附以治验和新方。该书与

2 The main content

The book consists of 24 volumes, which is divided into 8 categories, more than 260 articles in total, including menstruation regulation, numerous diseases, offspring praying, antenatal instruction, prenatal diagnosis, pregnancy, difficult delivery and puerperium. All dissertations have notes at the end of the article, and mostly with treating experience and new prescriptions. Compared with former works on obstetrics and

之前的妇产科著作比较有两个显著特点：

gynecology, this book has two distinct characteristics as follows:

(1) 提纲挈领

书中分类清楚，按照妇人的身体发育发展过程，以月经调理、造成月经不调的各种疾病、生育问题、胎教、妊娠期间的疾病、分娩过程中的常见疾病和产后的疾病等作为全书的论述线索，改变了之前的著述多“纲领散漫而无统”的状态，编排有序，条理井然。

(1) Being pertinent to the topic

Different from the former excursive works, this book is clearly-classified and quite well-organized in accordance with the process of woman's physical growth, mainly discussing menstruation regulation, various diseases caused by irregular menstruation, fertility problems, antenatal instruction, pregnancy, delivery and postpartum diseases, etc.

(2) 理论阐释全面

和之前的妇产科类著作不同，因作者中医基础功底扎实，通贯各中医理论知识，能运用脏腑经络等中医基础理论来阐述妇产科疾病，对各种妇产科病症较全面地用外感六淫、七情所伤、饮食不调、房事不节等致病因素进行分析，并着重用气血、冲任和脏腑理论解释病变机理，改变了以往著作中偏于罗列药方的做法。

(2) Comprehensive theory explanation

Different from previous works on obstetrics and gynecology, the author can apply basic theory of traditional Chinese medicine, like zang-fu organs and meridians, to elaborate on diseases of obstetrics and gynecology with his good grounding in the basic theories of traditional Chinese medicine. He can analyze various symptoms comprehensively with different pathogenic factors, such as six external etiological factors (wind, cold, summer-heat, dampness, dryness and fire), seven emotions (joy, anger, worry, overthinking, sorrow, fear and fright), irregular diet and excess of sexual intercourse, expounding mechanism of pathological changes with qi and blood, Ren vessels, and zang-fu theory instead of just listing formulas in the former books.

如对闭经一症能联系机体的脾肝病机，提出“滋其化源，其经自通”的观点；对结核引起的闭经主张用滋补药，反对泻下；并提出了在中医理论认识上重要的论点——“医风先医血，血行风自灭”的说法，成为后世治疗多种风证的重

For example, as for amenorrhea's association with body's pathogenesis of spleen and liver, he puts forward "menstruation adjusts itself by nourishing five zang-organs". For amenorrhea caused by tuberculosis, he proposes tonic drugs instead of purgative ones. And he suggests an important view on recognition of TCM theory—"regulating blood before curing wind syndromes, wind syndromes can be cured after blood circulation", which becomes the significant

要依据。

basis for curing wind syndromes in the later generations.

（3）内容丰富

（3）Rich content

书中内容极其丰富，如在调经门中有20篇论述，记述了有关月经的生理和病理特点，并分析了引起月经不调、闭经、痛经等月经异常变化的病因病机，确立了治法和具体方药；在众疾门中列有91篇论述，对一般常见的妇科疾病进行了讨论；在求嗣门列有10篇论述，阐述了导致不孕的原因主要有劳伤血气、经血闭涩、崩漏带下等三方面因素，并对早婚表示反对，认为男子30、女子20是结婚的适宜年龄；

The book is pretty rich in content. For instance, 20 articles in the category of "Menstruation Regulation" give an account of the physiological and pathological characteristics of menstruation, analyzing etiology and pathogenesis of abnormal changes of menstruation, such as irregular menstruation, amenorrhea and dysmenorrhea. Then, treatment and specific prescriptions are established. There are 91 articles in the category of "Numerous Diseases" discussing common gynecological diseases. In the category of "Infertility", 10 articles are listed to expound three factors that mainly cause the disease of infertility, such as internal injury of blood and qi due to overstrain, amenorrhea, metrorrhagia and metrostaxis, and gynecological disease, etc. Early marriage is opposed in this chapter, and the age of 20 for women and 30 for men are considered appropriate.

在胎教门中列有8篇论述，描述了妊娠时期各个阶段胎儿的发育情况；在候胎门中列有6篇论述，记载了有关妊娠的诊断，以及妊娠期间的禁忌药物如牛膝、三棱、大戟、巴豆、芫花、藜芦等，这些都已经被现代药理所证实；为便于学习者记诵，书中还列有孕妇禁忌歌；

There are 8 articles in the category of "Antenatal Instruction", describing fetus growth during all stages of pregnancy. In the category of "Fetus Diagnosis", 6 articles are listed to record the diagnosis of pregnancy and prohibited drugs during the period, such as twotoothed achyranthes root (niuxi), common buried rubber (sanleng), Peking euphorbia (daji), croton fruit (badou), lilac daphne flower bud (yuanhua), black false hellebore (lilu), which have been confirmed by modern pharmacology. For the convenience of reciting by learners, the book also lists songs on medicinal taboo for pregnant women.

在妊娠门中列有50篇论述，除叙述一般的孕期卫生如调节饮食、劳逸结合、个人卫生外，还重点讨论了妊娠期间特有的恶阻（妊娠呕吐）、子痫

In the category of "Pregnancy", 50 articles are included. Except for general description such as diet regulation, proper balance between work and rest and personal hygiene, this part mainly focuses on the discussion of diseases like vomiting during pregnancy, and eclamptism

（妊娠癫痫）等疾病；在产难门中有7篇论述，记述了各种难产和助产法；在产后门中有70篇论述，记载了产褥期的护理和感染情况等。此外书中还提供了不少行之有效的妇产科学方剂。

gravidarum (epilepsy of pregnancy). In the category of "Dystocia", there are 7 articles registering all kinds of difficult labours and delivery methods. In the category of "Postpartum", 70 articles are listed to record nursing and infection condition during puerperium. Additionally, the book also provides many effective prescriptions on obstetrics and gynecology.

三 学术价值

《妇人大全良方》在妇产科学方面是对前人成就及作者临床经验的总结，内容丰富，在理论上和实践上形成完整的体系，学术价值和实用价值很高，可以说是中国第一部完善的妇产科专著，为促进中国中医妇科学的发展做出了重要贡献，并长期为后世所应用。

3 Academic value

On obstetrics and gynecology, *A Complete Collection of Effective Prescriptions for Women* is the summary of former people's accomplishment and the author's clinical experience. It is of great academic and practical value with rich content and complete system both in theory and practice. The book is unarguably the first comprehensive monograph on obstetrics and gynecology in China, making significant contributions to the development of gynecology of TCM and has been applied since its compilation.

26 洗冤集录(Xiyuan Jilu)

Records of Washing Away of Wrong Cases

一 书籍简介

法医学是一门特殊的应用医学,中国早在汉代就有了关于法医检验的记载。随着人们对解剖知识的认识发展,宋朝又强化法制,推行了严厉的刑法,这些都促使法医学迅速发展。这期间最有价值并且长期影响国内外的法医学著作是成书于公元1247年的宋慈所著的《洗冤集录》。

宋慈(公元1186年—公元1249年)是进士出身,曾三次出任刑狱官,在长期的工作生涯中积累了丰富的司法经验,认为法医的检验在案件处理中具有非常重要的影响和作用,同时发现很多案件的错误判决多与法医检验的失误有关,因此他非常强调亲临现场勘验,审之又审,不敢懈怠。他总结了执法经验,并请教于医师,为避免错案、冤案的发生,精心撰写成《洗冤集录》一书,从而使中国古代法医学达到相当高的水平。

1 A brief introduction to the book

Forensic medicine is a special applied medicine. As early as the Han Dynasty, there appeared the record of forensic examination in China. With the the development of man's anatomical knowledge, legal system was enhanced in the Song Dynasty and strict criminal law was implemented, all of which promoted the rapid advancement of forensic medicine. During this time, the most valuable work on forensic medicine that had long-term impact both at home and abroad was *Records of Washing Away of Wrong Cases* (*Xiyuan Jilu*), which was written by Song Ci in 1247 A. D.

Song Ci (1186—1249 A. D.), origin of Jinshi (successful candidate in the highest imperial examination), had been served as a prison officer for three times. Thus, he had accumulated rich judiciary experience during his long-term career. He considered that forensic examination of doctors played key impact and role in case handling. Meanwhile, he found many wrong-judged cases were mostly caused by the fault of forensic examination, so that's why he emphasized that a forensic doctor must examine the case on the scene personally and repeatedly. By summing up his experience and asking doctors for advice, he compiled the book with elaborate care in order to avoid the misjudged cases and unjust cases, which made the Chinese ancient forensic medicine reach a higher level.

二 主要内容

《洗冤集录》全书共有5卷。卷1和卷2为检验总论，包括人体解剖、验伤、验尸、现场勘察等；卷3为各种机械性死伤原因的鉴别；卷4为可用于致死的各种毒物，包括有可能用于自杀或谋杀的动物、植物、矿物等各种毒品；卷5为各种急救与解毒方法，如用鸡蛋明矾灌救砒霜中毒、人工呼吸急救法等。

(1) 详细介绍了有关检验尸体的须知

书中介绍了当时关于检验尸体的法令以及各种检尸的方法和注意事项，系统阐述了法医学的尸体检查方法和各种死亡情况下的检查。强调法医必须迅速前往，即时亲验。验尸时切勿厌恶尸气，高坐远离，香烟蒸隔，任听他人禀报。书中也介绍了检验程序包括初检、复检，并详细规定各种验尸格式和方法，如先看头顶发际、耳窍、鼻孔、咽喉、肛门、阴道等可藏纳的地方，并要考虑光线明暗对尸体检验的影响，足见检验之精细。

(2) 区别不同的死亡原因

书中对各种原因引起的非正常死亡如自缢、勒死、溺死、他物手足伤死、自杀、杀伤、尸首异处、火死、汤泼死、服毒、受杖死、车轮碾死、雷震死、塌压

2 The main content

Records of Washing Away of Wrong Cases consists of five volumes. Volume 1 and volume 2 are general view of forensic examination, including autopsy, injury assessment, identification of corpse and spot investigation; volume 3 is about identification of causes for different mechanical casualty; volume 4 is about various lethal poisons, including animals, plants and minerals that can be used for suicide or murder; volume 5 is about different first-aid treatment and detoxification methods, for instance, artificial respiration or arsenic removal by copious flushings with alum and raw egg, etc.

(1) Detailed introduction to the notice about autopsy

The book introduces decree on autopsy at that time as well as its various methods and points for attention, giving a systematic explanation on forensic methods of postmortem examination and inspection under different circumstances of death. It is stressed that the coroner must immediately perform an autopsy in person and refrain from sitting comfortably behind a curtain of incense that masks the stench or letting his subordinates report to him for detesting the stench of corpses. The book also describes the procedures of examination, including initial examination and reexamina-tion, and stipulates examination methods and requirements, for example, the body parts where things can be hidden should be checked first, like hairline, external acoustic meatus, nostril, throat, anus and vagina. Besides, the influence of light on autopsy should be given consideration, which shows the meticulousness in examination.

(2) Distinction on different causes of death

The book records and describes abnormal death due to various causes, such as hanging oneself, strangulating, drowning, fatal injury, suicide, killing, dismembering, being burned by fire or boiling water, taking poison, flogging, crushed by rolling wheels, thundering, collapsing

死和针灸不当致死等都有记载和描述,并着重对许多死亡原因进行了区别或鉴定。

如提出四种机械性窒息死亡的方式——自缢、勒死、溺死和外物压塞口鼻死,并把自缢致死的绳套分为活套头、死套头、单系、十字缠绕系等,指出脚到地、膝跪地、卧于床等体位均可自缢而死,并指出牙齿出血是鉴别窒息死亡的一个重要证据;以伤口有无出血和肌肉组织的收缩情况,作为判断生前或死后损伤的依据,指出他杀的特点是死者手上常留有格斗伤痕,损伤部位多为本人所莫及;对焚死和焚尸区别指出凡生前被火烧死者,其尸口鼻内有烟灰,手脚皆蜷缩,若死后烧者,其人手足虽蜷缩,然口内无烟灰,这些见解都已为现代法医学所证实。

and improper acupuncturing. Differentiation and identification of many death causes are also stressed in this book.

For example, four ways to death by mechanical asphyxia are proposed in the book, including hanging oneself, strangulating, drowning and pressing upon mouth and nose with objects. Noose that used for hanging to death can be divided into slip knot, fast knot, single knot and cross knot. It points out some postures of hanging to death, such as standing, kneeling down and lying in bed; an important evidence to identify death by suffocation is teeth bleeding; injury suffered before or after death can be judged according to whether there is wound hemorrhage and contraction on muscle tissue; the characteristic of homicide is that the dead always have fighting scar left on their hands, and injured parts are mostly out of the reach of the dead. In terms of the distinction between burning to death and burning corpse after death, the dead with ashes in the mouth and nose are the ones burned before death with hands and feet huddled up. Otherwise, though hands and feet curling up, there are no ashes in the mouth of the one who is burned after death. All these views have been verified by modern forensic medicine.

(3) 记载了尸体现象

书中对法医检验过程中必然要遇到的尸体现象也有正确的认识,虽然没有直接提出"尸斑"的名称,但所描述的尸斑发生机理和分布特点非常精辟。如描述"凡死人,项后、背上、两肋、后腰、腿内、两臂上、两腿后、两腿肚子上下有微赤色";记述了尸体腐败的性状,影响腐败的条件,以及腐尸、常尸的检验区别。

(3) Record on postmortem phenomena

The book also shows correct recognition on postmortem phenomena that will appear certainly during the forensic examination. Though the term "livor mortis" is not mentioned directly, its occurrence mechanism and distribution characteristics are described pretty well, for example, the description of the phenomenon that "all the dead have slight-red color in the back neck, back, ribs, back waist, inner thigh, arms, back legs and two calves". It records the property of corrupted corpse, conditions for interrupting decay and the difference of examination between rotten corpse and fresh corpse.

三 学术价值

本书材料充实，内容丰富，论说简明，分析透彻，语言形象而生动，比较切合实际，故问世后便显示出不平凡的应用价值，数百年来一直被“官司检验奉为金科玉律”，成为死伤断狱的法典。后世法医著作大都以它为蓝本，并先后被译为朝、日、英、德、俄等多种文字流行于国际间，在世界法医史上有一定的影响和地位。

3 Academic value

After compilation, the book has shown its great application value for its abundant materials, rich content, concise explanation, thorough analysis, vivid and matter-of-fact language. For hundreds of years, it has always been "followed as an unalterable rule by lawsuit", becoming a code for the dead, the wound and criminal cases. As an original version for forensic books in the ages to come, it has been successively translated into many languages prevailing among international countries, such as Korea, Japan, English, German and Russia, exerting great influence in the world history of forensic medicine.

27 饮膳正要(Yinshan Zhengyao)

Principles of Correct Diet

一 书籍简介

从中国周朝时期开始,宫廷就设立有"食医",专门管理与饮食有关的医药问题。以后历代都有关于用饮食作为治疗手段的材料及专书出现,但是,讲究饮食营养,滋补身体,以达到强身养生的目的的书籍当以《饮膳正要》为最早。《饮膳正要》成书于公元1330年,是一部专门讲述食物营养、饮食卫生和食物疗法的书籍,是中医营养学的代表著作,为元代饮膳太医忽思慧所撰写,他在元朝曾任饮膳太医10余年,负责宫廷中的饮食调理、养生疗病诸事,加之他重视食疗与食补的研究与实践,因此有条件将元朝以前的宫廷食疗经验加以总结整理,并继承了前代的食疗学成就,汲取当时民间日常生活中的食疗经验,编撰成了营养学名著《饮膳正要》一书。

1 A brief introduction to the book

Since the beginning of the Zhou Dynasty (1046—256B. C.), dietitian has been set up in the court to specialize in administration on diet-related medical issues. Then, materials and specific books about taking diet as treatment measure have come into being during the past dynasties. However, *Principles of Correct Diet* (*Yinshan Zhengyao*) must be the earliest book aiming at body strengthening and health preservation by nutrition and nourishment. The book was compiled in 1330 A. D. and specialized in food nutrition, food hygiene and diet therapy. It was the representative work of traditional Chinese nutriology written by Hu Sihui, an imperial doctor in the Yuan Dynasty (1271—1368A. D.). He had been responsible for diet therapy and health nurturing for over a decade and paid special attention to the research and practice on both aspects, so it was available for him to summarize the court's experience of diet therapy before the Yuan Dynasty and compile the book by inheriting achievements of dietotherapy before the Yuan Dynasty and learning from the folk experience.

二 主要内容

《饮膳正要》共包括三卷,卷1讲述养生避忌、妊娠食

2 The main content

The book consists of three volumes. Volume 1 narrates taboo of health preserving, food restrictions for pregnant

忌、乳母食忌、饮酒避忌和各种珍奇食品的食谱等；分别叙述了汤、粉、羹、面、粥、馒头、烧饼等饭食，以及用蒸、炒、滑、炙、盐、熬等方法制成的菜肴。每种菜肴都说明其食疗效用、所用材料、调味品和烹调技术，卷2记载了各种汤煎等，并介绍了食物的四时所宜、用食疗治疗各种疾病、食物之间的相反和食物中毒等，阐述用于保健医疗的加药饮料与食品的配料及制作方法，寓养生治病于日常饮食，至今仍有参考价值，卷3记载了米谷类、鱼类和菜类等，对每种食品的性味与作用都逐一加以说明，大部分附有绘图，对加工成品简述其制法及疗效。

and lactating women, precautions of drinking, and some recipes of various rare foods. It describes respectively the diet such as soup, powder, thick soup, noodle, porridge, steamed buns and sesame seed cake, as well as dishes made by steaming, frying, sliding, roasting, salting, and boiling. The effectiveness of food therapy, ingredients, condiments and culinary techniques of every dish are also explained. Volume 2 covers various decoctions and introduces favorable foods for four seasons, disease treatment by diet therapy, counter-effects among food and food poisoning. It also narrates ingredients and processing methods of medicine-mixed beverage and food used for health care, which still have referrence value till today. Volume 3 registers grains, fish and vegetables, expounding nature and effect of each food with attached drawings. The processing methods and curative effect of manufactured products are also briefly introduced in this part.

（1）重视食品的医疗作用

该书继承了我国古代食、养、医结合的传统，全书的主旨在于“食补”，对每种食品都同时注意到它的食用、养生和医疗效果。作者从药物中选出无毒副作用可久食的补药，与饮食配合，调和五味，供调养身体所用。如苦豆汤具有“补下元，理腰膝，顺气”的治疗功效；生地黄烧鸡具有“治腰背疼痛，骨髓虚损，身重气乏”的效果；鲫鱼羹具有“治脾胃虚弱，泻痢久不愈者，食之大效”的作用。书中展示的食物既是鲜美可口的佳肴，又是

(1) Emphasizing the medical function of food

Inheriting the Chinese tradition that integrates food, nourishment and medicine in ancient times, the book aims at “dietary cure”, that is, paying attention to edible function, health preservation and medical effect of each food at the same time. From all drugs, the author selects tonifying ones with no toxicity or side effects for long-time taking, which can be used for nursing body if they match with diet. For example, sophora alopecuroides decoction is good for “nourishing the primary qi in the lower body, restraining the pain in the waist and knees, and promoting the circulation of qi”, chicken cooked with unprocessed rehmannia root for “treating backache, deficiency of bone marrow, and heavy body and exhausting qi”, crucian soup's effectiveness for “curing weakness in spleen and stomach, diarrhea dysentery for a long time”. The food shown in the book is not only delicious dishes, but also

强壮身体、延年益寿、预防和治疗疾病的良药。

good medicines that help to strengthen body, prolong life, prevent and cure diseases.

(2) 提倡饮食卫生

书中除了说明各种饮食的烹调方法外,还特别注重饮食与营养卫生的关系,这是别的一般食谱中所没有的。它从健康人的实际饮食需要出发,以正常人膳食标准立论,制定了一套饮食卫生法则。书中提倡先饥后食,勿令食饱,先渴而饮,饮勿令过;不可饱食而卧,尤其夜间不可多食用,勿食不洁或变质之物,不可大醉,食毕宜用温水漱口,睡前刷牙等。此外还提到了有关食物中毒的防治,列举了许多有效的解毒方法。

(2) Advocating dietetic hygiene

In addition to the explanation for cooking methods, the book also attaches importance to the relations between diet and nutrition hygiene, which is unique compared with other general recipes. Starting from the dietary needs of healthy people and dietary standards for the normal, a series of rules for dietetic hygiene has been set up. The book advises people not to eat to fullness, not to drink too much after thirst, not to lie after eating too much, especially not to eat excessively in the midnight, not to eat unclean or rotten food, not to be drunk, to gargle with warm water after meal, to brush teeth before going to bed, etc. Besides, it also mentions the prevention and treatment relating to food poisoning and lists many effective detoxifying methods.

(3) 记载了汉蒙民族的丰富食物

书中将汉蒙民族的食物兼收并蓄,所述用料兽品以羊、牛居先,次及马、驼、鹿、猪等,奇珍异馔中用羊肉制成者占十分之七。该书记载药膳方和食疗方非常丰富,特别注重阐述各种饮食物的性味与滋补作用,还增补有一些以前药物书籍所未曾记载的药物及其功效。

(3) Registering rich food of the Mongolian and Han nationalities

The book also covers the food of the Mongolian and Han nationalities. Among the mentioned food ingredients most of them are from sheep and cow, and some from horse, camel, deer and pig, etc. Mutton accounts for 70% among rare food. Plentiful formulas of herbal diet and food therapy are registered in this book, including the nature, flavor and nourishment of different food. Also, some medicines and their effects that have never been recorded in the former medical books are supplemented.

三 学术价值

《饮膳正要》在我国古代营养学发展史上占有重要的地位。它既是现存最完整的古代

3 Academic value

The book occupies an important place in the Chinese history of ancient nutriology. It is not only the most complete monograph on diet hygiene and diet therapy in the

饮食卫生和食治疗法专书，也是一部现存最早的古代食谱。这是一部融合蒙汉两族饮食文化的文献，内容涉及现代营养卫生学的各主要方面，交织反映了当时饮食医药文化的成就。总之《饮膳正要》是一部很有价值的科学著作，对传播和发展我国的卫生保健知识做出了积极的贡献。

ancient times, but also the earliest existing one on recipes in China. The document which integrates the diet culture of the Mongolian and Han nationalities involves the main aspects on modern nutrition hygiene, interlacedly reflecting the achievements of diet and medicine culture at that time. In short, it is a scientific work with great value, making positive contributions to the spread and development of knowledge about Chinese health care.

28 敖氏伤寒金镜录(Aoshi Shanghan Jinjing Lu)

Ao's Golden Mirror Records for Cold Damage

一 书籍简介

中医学中的舌诊是颇具特色的诊断方法,在《内经》、《伤寒杂病论》中均重视舌的形态、质地和舌苔在诊断疾病上的意义。《敖氏伤寒金镜录》是我国现存的第一部图文并茂的舌诊专书。作者姓敖,名字信息不全,他对舌诊进行了详细的研究,并将临床察舌辨证的经验总结而写成该书。此书写成以后因当时信息传播条件有限,未能广为流行,以至现在已看不到原来的版本了。好在当时有个叫杜清碧的人,发现了这本书以后自己动手绘了24幅舌象图,与原书12幅图合为36幅,于公元1341年印刷出版。我们现在看到的《敖氏伤寒金镜录》就是经杜清碧增补的版本。

1 A brief introduction to the book

Observing the tongue is a special diagnostic method in traditional Chinese medicine. The shape, texture and coating of the tongue are of great importance to the disease diagnosis, which has been mentioned in *Internal Classic* and *Treatise on Cold Damage and Miscellaneous Diseases*. *Ao's Golden Mirror Records for Cold Damage* (*Aoshi Shanghan Jinjing Lu*) is the first existing book in China specialized in tongue diagnosis with vivid illustrations. The author, with his surname Ao, made a detailed research on tongue diagnosis and compiled the book through the summary on clinical experience of observation and differentiation. The original version is unavailable now because the information communication at that time was too limited to make the book be spread widely. Fortunately, a person named Du Qingbi drew 24 pictures of the tongue characteristics by himself after finding the original version, and then, by integrating with 12 pictures in the original one, he printed and published the book in 1341 A. D. with 36 pictures in total. The existing book is just the version supplemented by Du Qingbi.

二 主要内容

《敖氏伤寒金镜录》中主要讨论了伤寒的舌诊,列有舌象图12幅,后经杜清碧增补了24图,合为36种彩色图

2 The main content

The book mainly deals with the tongue diagnosis of cold damage. Among 36 color pictures, 24 particularly discuss the tongue coating, 4 analyze the tongue body and 8 discuss concurrently on both the coating and body. As the

谱,其中有24图专论舌苔,4图论舌质,8图兼论舌苔和舌质。图中所记载的舌色有淡、红、青3种;舌面变化有红刺、红点、裂纹等;苔色有白、黄、灰、黑四种;苔质有干、滑、涩、刺、偏、全等描述。该书基本对常见的主要病理舌象都作以描述,每图配有文字说明,并结合脉象阐述所主证候的病因病机、治法和预后判断等。该书以伤寒疾病为主,也涉及一些内科疾病以及其他疾病。这本关于舌诊的专门著作对于临床诊断中舌诊的应用具有重要的指导意义。

pictures shows, the color of the tongue may be pale, red and blue; the changes on the surface of the tongue include red prickle, red spots and cracks; the four colors of the coating are white, yellow, gray and black; and the coating texture can be described as dry, slippery, rough, prickled, deviated and greasy. Above all, the main tongue manifestations are narrated with illustrations, and the main syndromes' etiology, pathogenesis, treatment, and prognosis are expounded according to the pulse condition. Apart from the cold damage, the book also involves some internal and other diseases. As an monograph on tongue diagnosis, it plays a significant guiding role in the clinical application of tongue diagnosis.

三 学术价值

历代医家对该书都有很高的评价,如明朝的著名医家薛己评论该书"专以舌色视病……开卷昭然,一览俱在",并认为该书的理论思想立足于医圣仲景之道,内容丰富而昭然揭示医理,简单明了而得舌诊的要领,对于临床诊断具有不可忽略的影响。后来该书曾经在日本广为流传,对日本的汉方医学诊法产生了深刻的影响。《敖氏伤寒金镜录》作为舌诊学的开山之作,不仅奠定了舌诊学的基础,而且在理论标识、方法创新及临床实用等方面均有独到的贡献,在中国舌诊学史上具有重要的地位。

3 Academic value

Doctors through the ages spoke highly of the book. For example, Xue Ji, a famous physician in the Ming Dynasty, made a comment that the book "examining disease according to the tongue color, ... which are all clearly described in the book". He also considered that the theory of the book is based on the doctrine of medical saint Zhang Zhongjing. With its rich content to reveal the medical knowledge and brief expression to show the core of tongue diagnosis, the book has produced an ineligible effect on clinical diagnosis. It also has been spread widely in Japan afterwards, bringing impressive influence on its diagnostic methods of Chinese medicine. As a pioneering work, *Ao's Golden Mirror Records for Cold Damage* is of great importance in the history of tongue diagnosis because it not only lays a foundation for tongue diagnosis, but also makes unique contributions to theory identification, method innovation and clinical application.

29 世医得效方(Shiyi Dexiao Fang)

Effective Prescriptions Handed Down from Generations of Physicians

一 书籍简介

《世医得效方》是一部内容涉及中医内、外、妇、儿、骨伤、五官等各科疾病的方书，对骨伤科证治尤多发挥，是由元朝危亦林(公元1277年—公元1347年)编撰，刊行于公元1345年。危亦林出身世医之家，从小勤奋好学，博览医经，并深得家传，对内、外、妇、儿、眼、骨伤、口齿咽喉等科均有研究，尤其擅长骨伤科。他学识渊博，医术高超，在长期临床实践中，有感于古代的医方浩瀚如烟，不方便检索应用，于是依按古方并参照家传的方剂内容，编成了《世医得效方》。

1 A brief introduction to the book

Effective Prescriptions Handed Down from Generations of Physicians (*Shiyi Dexiao Fang*) is a medical formulary concerning diseases of different sections, such as internal medicine, surgery, gynecology, pediatrics, orthopedics, and otolaryngology, particularly specialized in orthopedics. It was compiled by Wei Yilin (1277—1347 A. D.) and published in 1345 A. D. in the Yuan Dynasty. Born in the family that had practiced medicine for generations, Wei worked hard and read widely on the medical knowledge when he was a little child, so he got what had been handed down in his family. He studied respectively on internal medicine, surgery, gynecology, pediatrics, ophthalmology, orthopedics, otolaryngology and other branches of TCM, especially was good at orthopedics. During the long term of clinical practice, confronted with inconvenience for search and application among the numerous prescriptions in ancient times, Wei finished the compilation of the book by referring to the old prescriptions and family inherited ones.

二 主要内容

全书共分20卷。卷1至卷10为大方脉杂医科，卷11至卷12为小方脉科，卷13为风科，卷14至卷15为产科兼妇人杂病科，卷16为眼科，卷17为口齿兼咽喉科，卷18为正骨兼金镞科，卷19为疮肿

2 The main content

The book consists of 20 volumes, among which, the section of miscellaneous diseases for adult is introduced from volume 1 to volume 10; the section for children covers volume 11 and 12; volume 13 is the section of wind; volume 14 and 15 deal with obstetrics and miscellaneous diseases of women; volume 16, 17, 18 and 19 are respectively the section of ophthalmology, dentistry and stomatology, as well

科，卷20为附篇，附有养生内容。书中按照证候和方药分类，纲目分明，具有较高的学术价值，尤其对骨伤科的贡献最大。

as pharyngeal and laryngeal, the section of bone setting and metal-inflicted wound, and the section of sores and wounds; volume 20 is the attachment to the book with the content of health preservation. Classified with syndromes and prescriptions, the book is of great academic value with clear outline, especially making the biggest contribution to orthopedics.

(1) 骨折部位诊断分类的进步

作者将四肢骨折和关节脱位归纳为"六出臼，四折骨"。前者是指肩、肘、腕、髋、膝、踝六大关节脱位，后者则指肱骨、前臂骨、股骨、胫腓骨四大长骨骨折。这种说法反映出当时医学对全身主要的骨折、关节脱位都已有较深刻的认识。作者还强调在诊断骨折的时候，必须要触摸辨别骨折移动的方向。书中首次记载了肩关节有前上方脱位和盂下脱位两大类型，并指出足踝部骨折脱位有内翻和外翻的区别，这些都大大丰富了中医骨伤科的诊断。

(1) Advancement in diagnosis classification of fracture locations

The author sums up the limb fracture and joint dislocation as "six dislocations, four bone fractures", reflecting an profound recognition of medical science at that time to the main fracture and dislocation on the whole body. The former refers to dislocations of six joints such as shoulder, elbow, wrist, pelvis, knee and ankle; the latter refers to fracture of four long bones including humerus, forearm bones, femur, and tibia and fibula. Also, the author emphasizes that doctors must touch the fracture to find out which direction it is moving. The book firstly records that shoulder joint dislocation includes anterior dislocation and infraglenoid dislocation, and points out that there are differences between inversion and eversion on the fracture dislocation of the foot and ankle, which all greatly enrich the TCM diagnosis of orthopedics and traumatology.

(2) 骨折脱位整复法的创新

在骨折脱位的治疗方面，危亦林有许多创新和发明。如首次采用悬吊复位法治疗脊椎骨折。他认为脊椎骨折往往引起压缩性骨折，单靠手法整复难以复位，因此必须要用悬吊的方法复位。具体地：

"须用软绳从脚吊起，坠下身直，其骨使自归窠，未直则未归窠，须要坠下待其骨直

(2) Innovation in reduction therapy of fracture dislocation

Wei makes lots of innovations in the treatment of fracture dislocation. For the first time, for example, he treats spine fracture by suspension with soft rope. He believes that spine fracture tends to trigger compression fracture, which cannot be reset only by reduction manipulation, but suspension.

"The feet are lifted by soft rope and the body is straightly suspended, thus, making its bone reset on the right place of the body, so that's why suspension must be done for straight bone reduction", which emphasizes that only

归窠”，强调伸直脊椎才能复位。这种悬吊复位的方法，不仅是我国伤科史上的重大发明，也是世界医学史上的创举（英国医生 Davis 在 1927 年才应用悬吊复位法治疗脊椎骨折）。对肩关节脱位的治疗方法已经不需要医者的牵引和旋转，仅借助患者自己的身体下坠力而达到复位目的。对肘部脱臼骨折，除用手法复位外，还提出用夹板外固定。对足踝关节骨折复位则主张应用牵引、反向复位的方法。

with straight spine can reduction be resulted. This suspension method is not only a great invention in the history of department of traumatology, but also a pioneering work in the history of world medicine (Davis, an English doctor who did not apply the suspension method to treat spine fracture until 1927). Instead of doctors' applying traction and rotation to treat dislocation of the shoulder joint, the patients, therefore can also get reduction by their own physical dropping force. For fractures or dislocations of elbow, Wei suggests external fix with splints except for manual reposition. He recommends applying traction and reverse reset in fracture reduction of foot and ankle joints.

（3）动静结合的治疗思想

作者在书中十分强调骨折固定和活动相结合的原则，强调骨折脱位在复位后需要适当活动以防关节粘连，如肘、膝盖关节复位固定后“不可放定”，而要经常曲直加以活动锻炼，否则此处很容易因为活动少而关节粘连，造成以后的功能受限、不能活动等遗留问题。

(3) Therapy thought combining dynamics and statics

The author gives much emphasis on the combination of the fix and activity of fracture, and on the appropriate activity needed for preventing joint adhesion after reposition of fracture dislocation. After the reduction fix of knee joint, for example, rather than "static-remaining", knee should be frequently bent and straightened with dirigation. Otherwise, it would be easy to cause joint adhesion because of the lack of activity, bringing about remaining problems such as limited functions and no movements.

（4）麻醉术在骨折脱位整复中的正确使用

在《世医得效方》中作者首次把使用曼陀罗的全身麻醉术用于骨科临床。危亦林特别重视麻醉术在骨折脱位治疗中的应用，常选用曼陀罗、草乌等作为麻醉药物，认为“治伤损骨节不归窠者，以此麻之，然后用手整顿”；“诸骨碎、骨折、脱臼者，与服麻药二钱，和酒调下，

(4) Correct use of anesthesia technology during the reduction of fracture dislocation

In the book, general anesthesia technology that uses jimsonweed (mantuoluo) is first applied to clinical orthopedics. Wei pays particular attention to the application of anesthesia in treating fracture dislocation. He often selects jimsonweed and kusnezoff monkshood root (caowu) as anesthetic drugs. He advocates that "to treat the dislocation of injured bone with narcosis before manual manipulation"; "to treat broken bone, fracture or dislocation by mixing anesthetic drugs of 2 qian(a unit of weight in ancient China,

麻到不知痛处,或用刀割开,或剪去骨锋者,以手整顿骨节,归原端正,用夹夹定";并指出必须按患者年龄、体质、出血等具体情况决定麻醉药的剂量,这些要求与现代医学麻醉原则基本相同。

在欧洲19世纪中叶发明乙醚等麻醉药之前,日本外科医生曾于1805年使用曼陀罗作为手术麻醉药,被誉为世界麻醉史上的佳话和先例。其实此法不仅比《世医得效方》晚了460余年,比公元1146年窦材的《扁鹊心书》中用曼陀罗麻醉的记载更晚了650多年。可见这些有关麻醉药物的记载,应当是世界麻醉史上最早的文献。

1 qian equals to 5 grams) with spirit, it would be too numb for the patients to feel painful after taking it, then use knife to cut the sharp part of the bone for joint reset and clamp fix with hands". Furthermore, details about the dosage of anesthetic drugs are decided by ages, constitution and hemorrhage of patients. All these requests are basically the same for anesthesia as the rules of the modern medicine.

Prior to the invention of anaesthetic such as ether in the mid-19th century in Europe, jimsonweed was used as anesthetic in operation by Japanese surgeons in 1805, which was reputed to be a legacy and precedent in the history of anesthesia. As a matter of fact, the practice was not only over 460 years later than that in *Effective Formulae Handed Down for Generations*, but also even over 650 years later than that in *Bian Que Heart Book*, written by Dou Cai, who also recorded narcosis with jimsonweed in 1146 A. D. Thus, it is obvious that these records related to drugs for anesthesia should be the earliest literature in the history of anesthesia in the world.

三 学术价值

危亦林在学术上造诣很深,且敢于突破"传子不传女"的传统观念,把五世祖传秘方公之于世,这种精神十分可贵。他反对墨守成规,强调对古代成方必须通晓其要领,融会贯通,灵活运用,因此《世医得效方》中反映了作者丰富的临症经验和善于化裁古方的创新思想。该书对于中医学的骨伤科诊断、治疗等方面都具有重大的贡献,所创立的悬吊复位法成为骨伤科医学史上的创举。

3 Academic value

Wei was very accomplished academically. His spirit was very precious because he dared to break through the traditional concept that "impart knowledge only to sons", and made a secret recipe handed down for five generations from his ancestors known by the general public. He objected to obeying the old rules and emphasized on thorough understanding of core meaning of the ancient prescriptions. Thus, the book embodies the author's rich clinical experience and innovative thought of revising ancient prescriptions. Besides significant contributions to TCM traumatology and orthopedics in diagnosis and treatment, the suspension created by the book becomes a pioneering undertaking in the medical history of traumatology and orthopedics.

30 救荒本草(Jiuhuang Bencao)

Materia Medica for Famine Relief

一 书籍简介

《救荒本草》是明朝早期的一部植物图谱,作者朱橚(公元1360年—公元1425年)是明朝开国皇帝朱元璋的第五个儿子。他"好学能文,留心民事",为了能在遇到荒年时帮助百姓渡过饥饿,在王府中建立了一个专门的植物园,栽培研究各种植物。他征集了400余种植物种植在园内,包括很多野生植物在内,亲自进行种植观察,召集画工绘制植物的图,描述植物的花、实、根、干、皮、叶等形态,总结了414种植物的名称、产地、形态、性味、烹调法等并编辑成《救荒本草》,重在介绍可食用的野生植物,开辟了食源,增强了民众抗灾能力。该书于公元1406年刊行,是我国历史上最早的一部以救荒为宗旨的农学、植物学专著书,对植物资源的利用、加工炮制等方面也做了全面的总结,对我国植物学、农学、医药学等科学的发展都有一定影响。

1 A brief introduction to the book

Materia Medica for Famine Relief (*Jiuhuang Bencao*) is a plant atlas, whose author Zhu Su (1360—1425 A. D.) is the fifth son of Zhu Yuanzhang, the first emperor in the Ming Dynasty. He was keen on study, good at liberal arts and concerned about civil affairs. For helping the mass get through starvation when confronting with the famine, he built a specialized botanical garden to cultivate and study various plants in his imperial mansion. He accumulated more than 400 plants that include many wild ones in the garden, made planting and observation by himself. Painters were called together to draw pictures of these plants and described their forms, such as flower, fruit, root, trunk, bark, and leaf. Totally, 414 kinds of plants were collected and compiled into the book, including their names, origins, forms, nature, flavor and cookery. Particularly, the author gave priority to the introduction of edible wild plants, exploring the source of food and enhancing people's disaster-combat ability. The book, published in 1406, is the earliest monograph of agronomy and botany aiming to the relief of famines in China. It reaches a comprehensive conclusion on the utilization and processing of plant resources, making an impact on the development of botany, agronomy and medicine.

二 主要内容

全书分上、下两卷，共记载植物414种，每种都配有精美的木刻插图。其中出自历代药物学著作的有138种，新增276种，分为草类245种、木类80种、米谷类20种、果类23种、菜类46种等。与大多数药物书比较，该书具有的特点是：① 植物之分类除按草、木、米、谷、果、菜区分为六大部分，还依据植物的可食用部分区分为叶可食、实可食、叶实可食、根可食、根叶可食、根实可食、根笋可食、根花可食、花可食、花叶可食、花实可食、茎可食、笋可食、笋实可食等14类；② 所收载的植物绝大部分是人们日常不食用者；③ 每种植物除记载名称、生产环境、形态、性味外，另辟有“救饥”一栏以说明该植物可供采集的部分、加工、消除毒性异味及调制食用方法；④ 书中有文字说明也有插图，以方便辨认植物并采集。

2 The main content

The book can be divided into two volumes with 414 varieties of plants, each with a fine woodcut. Among them, 138 are originated from pharmacology works of past dynasties and 276 are added, falling into 245 herbs, 80 trees, 20 grains, 23 fruits and 46 vegetables. Compared with most works of materia medica, this book is characterized by the following 4 points:①in addition to the classification of herb, tree, grain, fruit and vegetable, plants are also divided into 14 varieties according to their edible parts such as edible leaves or fruits, edible leaves and fruits, edible roots, edible roots and leaves, edible roots and fruits, edible roots and bamboo, edible roots and flowers, edible flowers, edible flowers and leaves, edible flowers and fruits, edible stems or bamboo, edible bamboo and fruit, etc. ②plants collected in the book are mostly non-edible food in people's daily lives. ③except for registered names, habitats, shapes, nature and favor, the column “Starvation Relief” is created to show that all plants have parts available for collection, processing, toxicity and ill-smelling elimination and how to make and eat them; ④for the convenience of recognizing and gathering plants, there are both words and illustrations attached to the book.

三 学术价值

《救荒本草》既是一本食、药两用的植物学著作，也是一本植物学图谱，在植物学与农学、医学方面均有较大价值。此书出版后在明朝就曾多次翻刻，在国内和国外都产生了一定影响。约在17世纪末，

3 Academic value

Materia Medica for Famine Relief is not only a work on botany specialized in food and medicine, but also a plant atlas with great value in botany, agronomy and medicine. Since its publication, the book had been printed for many times in the Ming Dynasty. It is making certain influence both at home and abroad. At the end of 17th century, the

《救荒本草》流传到了日本，当时的日本自然灾害频繁，《救荒本草》以其"救荒"的意义引起了日本学者的关注，并对该书内容进行多次出版研究。

book was introduced to Japan. Plagued by natural disasters, Japanese scholars turned their eyes upon the literature and its meaning of "famine relief", and studied the book, making it printed for many times.

31 普济方(Puji Fang)

Formulary of Universal Relief

一 书籍简介

《普济方》是明朝时期的一部方剂书籍,也是我国古代最大的一部方书。该书是由明朝的开国皇帝朱元璋的第五个儿子朱橚(公元1361年—公元1425年)主持并组织人执笔汇编而成。朱橚本人一直很喜欢研究医药学,平时很注意收集古今的方剂,为了编写《普济方》而组织人员收集了大量资料,书中共收集药方61 739首,集15世纪以前中医学方书之大成。该书刊行于1406年,由于当时出版数量较少,而该书又比较实用,《普济方》在当时十分珍贵,所以不少人辗转传抄。但是该书的初刻本已经散佚,后来的收藏也都残缺不全,所幸全书在清朝的《四库全书》中收载保存。

1 A brief introduction to the book

Formulary of Universal Relief (*Puji Fang*) is a book on formula in the Ming Dynasty, It is also the biggest medical formulary in ancient times of China. The compilation of the book was hosted and organized by Zhu Su (1361—1425A. D.), who was the fifth son of Zhu Yuanzhang (the first emperor of the Ming Dynasty). He was always keen on studying medicine and used to collect formulas that ever existed. For the compilation of the book, he arranged compilers to accumulate plentiful materials, thus the book epitomizing medical formulary before 15th century with 61,739 formulas in total. The book, published in 1406, was quite practical and of great value. A lot of people made private copies because of its few publication. Fortunately, the complete version was preserved in *Complete Collection of the Four Treasures* of the Qing Dynasty though its primary edition had been lost and collected versions later were also incomplete.

二 主要内容

全书原为169卷,后经《四库全书》改编为426卷,初本尚有插图239幅。全书大致分为12部分,卷1—卷5为

2 The main content

Originally, the book consists of 169 volumes and then was reedited into 426 volumes in *Complete Collection of the Four Treasures* with 239 illustrations in the primary version. The whole book can be roughly divided into 12 parts:

方脉，卷 6—卷 12 为运气，卷 13—卷 43 为脏腑，卷 44—卷 86 为五官，卷 87—卷 250 为内科杂病，卷 251—卷 267 为杂治，卷 268—卷 272 为杂录和符禁，卷 273—卷 315 为外伤科，卷 316—卷 357 为妇科，卷 358—卷 408 为儿科，卷 409—卷 424 为针灸，卷 425—卷 426 为本草。内容包括了方脉总论、药性总论、五运六气、脏腑总论、脏腑各论（按人身头面、体表、五官、口齿和内部脏腑器官分述各种病候）、伤寒杂病（包括各种急性、慢性传染病与内科疾病）、外科、骨科、妇科、儿科、针灸等。每种病症都有论有方，除记载药物与针灸治疗方法，还介绍了按摩、导引等治疗经验。整体书中内容编次条理清晰，内容十分丰富。

volumes 1 to 5 cover medical formula and pulse condition, volumes 6 to 12 cover qi distribution, volumes 13 to 43 cover zang-fu organs, volumes 44 to 86 cover five sense organs, volumes 87 to 250 cover miscellaneous diseases in internal medicine, volumes 251 to 267 cover mixed treatment, volumes 268 to 272 cover miscellanea and abracadabra, volumes 273 to 315 cover traumatic surgery, volumes 316 to 357 cover gynecology, volumes 358 to 408 cover pediatrics, volumes 409 to 424 cover acupuncture and moxibustion, volumes 425 to 426 cover materia medica. It includes general treatise on medical formula and pulse condition, medical speciality, five movements and six climates, zang-fu organs, special viscera (discussion on various diseases according to body, head, face, body surface, five sense organs, teeth and internal zang-fu organs), febrile and miscellaneous diseases (including acute diseases, chronic infectious diseases and internal diseases), surgery department, orthopedics department, pediatrics and acupuncture and moxibustion department, etc. Every syndrome has its own analysis and prescription. Besides the record of medicines and methods of acupuncture treatment, it also includes the introduction of treatment experience such as medical massage and physical and breathing exercises. As a whole, the book is clear in its order of arrangement and rich in content.

三 学术价值

《普济方》是一本十分实用的方书，搜罗广泛，资料丰富，不仅在中医方剂史上有着重要价值，同时也保存了明朝以前的大量医学文献，为后人提供了宝贵的资料，例如明朝著名的药物学家李时珍在编著《本草纲目》过程中，虽然浏览参考的各种文献多达 800 余种，但明朝以前的不少失传或罕见的医籍李时珍未能亲

3 Academic value

Formulary of Universal Relief is a practical medical formulary with rich materials. It is of significant value in the history of TCM that formulas and numerous medical documents before the Ming Dynasty are also collected, bringing precious materials to the later generations. In the Ming Dynasty, for example, a famous pharmacologist Li Shizhen looked up to more than 800 references during his compilation of *Compendium of Materia Medica*, but he failed to touch many lost or rare medical classics before the Ming Dynasty. Fortunately, he got many sources from *Formulary*

睹，幸得以从《普济方》转引。该书中广博的资料除收录了历代方书外，还兼收史传、杂说、道藏、佛典中的有关内容，为我们保留了许多佚失的珍贵材料。

of Universal Relief. The book embraces both medical formulary of the past dynasties and relevant contents on historical records, various opinions, Taoist sutra as well as Buddhist scripture, reserving for us plenty of lost valuable materials.

32 本草纲目(Bencao Gangmu)

Compendium of Materia Medica

一 书籍简介

《本草纲目》是明清时期最重要的综合性本草,是我国古代最伟大的药学著作,该书集古代本草学之大成,是16世纪以前药物学的全面总结,分类科学、内容丰富,在世界科技史上占有重要地位。作者李时珍(公元1518年—1593年)字东壁,号濒湖山人,出身医学世家,14岁考中秀才,后科考不第,致力于医药,渐有声誉,并曾被推荐到太医院任职。因李时珍认为历代有关药物的著作存在谬误遗漏等众多问题而决心重编,从公元1552年至公元1578年,历时27年,三易其稿,撰写成《本草纲目》这本药物学巨著。

1 A brief introduction to the book

Compendium of Materia Medica is the most important comprehensive work on traditional Chinese materia medica during the Ming and Qing dynasties and the greatest pharmaocological work in ancient China. It epitomizes the pharmaceutical achievements and developments before the 16th century, occupying an important position in the world history of science and technology with its scientific classification and wide-ranging content. The author Li Shizhen (1518—1593A. D.), courtesy name Dongbi, who styled himself as *Bin Hu Shan Ren*, was born into a medical family. He passed the imperial examination at the country level when he was 14, but failed in the higher level later. Thereafter, he began to dedicate himself to Chinese medicine and once had been recommended to work in Imperial Academy of Medicine for the higher reputation he had earned. Since Li thought that there were lots of errors and omissions in the ancient works on drugs, he determined to re-edit the book. It took Li 27 years (1552—1578 A. D.) to complete the book, after modifying for three times.

二 主要内容

作者"渔猎群书,搜罗百氏"著成此书,书中有作者大量的实地观察和核实,并且作者亲自请教于药农、樵夫、猎人、皮匠、渔民等人以纠正以往药物学著作中的错误。全

2 The main content

Drawing reference from a wide range of works, the compendium contains extensive knowledge and large amount of empirical observation and verification. Furthermore, the author, in person, rectified many past mistakes by consulting medicinal herb growers, woodcutters, hunters, cobblers and fishermen. The book is a 52-volume compilation, including

书共有52卷:第1—第2卷为总论,介绍药物学的气味阴阳、升降浮沉、用药禁忌等知识;第3—第4卷主要列举临床各科的百余种疾病和常用药;第5—第52卷为具体的药物各论。书中共记载药物1 892种,附有方剂11 096首,配有插图1 000余幅,总计190万字。

one thousand plus pictures, written in about 1.9 million Chinese words. Volumes 1 to 2 are the general introduction to the knowledge of materia medica, such as qi and flavor, yin and yang, ascending and descending, floating and sinking, and taboos for drugs usage. Volumes 3 to 4 mainly introduce hundreds of diseases and commonly-used drugs in clinical practice, and volumes 5 to 52 give detailed descriptions of individual drugs. In all, the book records 1,892 kinds of medicines with 11,096 prescriptions.

(1) 提出了当时最先进的药物分类法

李时珍在《本草纲目》中对药物分类按照"从微至巨"、"从贱至贵"的原则,即从无机到有机、从低等到高等,基本上符合进化论的观点,因而是当时世界上最先进的分类法,并且按照"物以类从"而列出纲目总司药物的种类,便于寻觅查阅。书中共以水、火、土、金石、草、谷、菜、果、木、服器、虫、鳞、介、禽、兽、人等16部为纲,60类为目,基本上达到了纲目清晰的程度。

(1) Proposing the most advanced medicinal classification

In accordance with the principle of "from micro to giant, from humble to noble", Li classifies the medicine from inorganic to organic materials and lower to higher level. This classification method was the most advanced in the world at that time as it basically conforms to the theory of evolution. And for convenience of reference, the book further classifies medicines into 16 categories and 60 items according to the principle of "like attracts like". Clear and detailed descriptions are given under the following 16 categories: water, fire, earth, metal and stone , grasses, grains, vegetables, fruits, wood, clothes and utensils, insects and worms, animals with scale, animals with shell, poultry, beasts, and parts of human body which can be used as medicine.

(2) 系统地记述了各种药物的知识

《本草纲目》对每种药物的记述,包括校正、释名、集解、辨疑、正误、修治、气味、主治、发明、附录、附方等项。从药物的名称、历史、形态、鉴别到采集、加工、功效、方剂等,叙述甚详,尤其是发明这项,主要是李时珍对药物观察、研

(2) Describing various medicines systematically

The compendium gives exhaustive descriptions about each drug, including revision, names and explanations, paraphrase, exegesis, recognition, correction, processing method, flavor and taste, indication, invention, appendix and relevant prescriptions. It records and describes the name, origin, appearance, identification of drugs, as well as collection, processing, efficacy and prescriptions in detail. Particularly the part of invention mainly comes from Li's observation, research on drugs, and new discoveries

究以及实际应用的新发现和新经验，这就更加丰富了本草学的知识。

and experience of practical application, which greatly enriches knowledge of herbalism.

(3) 纠正了一些反科学的见解和错误内容

(3) Rectifying some anti-science opinions and wrong content

李时珍通过科学的总结，批判了以往古人所记载的服食水银、雄黄等可以长生不老的说法，纠正了一些反科学的错误观点，同时对历代药物著作中的错误作了修正，如把以前错误地认为是植物果实的五倍子更正为虫巢。

Through scientific conclusion, Li rectifies and criticizes some anti-science misconceptions, such as the view that people who take mercury and realgar (xionghuang) can be immortal. At the same time, he amends some mistakes in the medicinal works throughout the ages, such as revising gallnut to insect nest, which was wrongly regarded as fruit of plants.

(4) 丰富了世界科学宝库

(4) Enriching the world's science treasure

《本草纲目》不仅对药物学做了详细记载，同时对人体生理、病理、疾病的症状、卫生预防等方面作了不少正确的叙述，而且还综合了大量的科学资料，在植物学、动物学、矿物学、物理学、化学、农学、天文、气象等许多方面有着广泛的论述。如在动物学方面对鸵鸟的描述；在矿物学方面对石油的产地与性状的记述；在物理学方面记载了借助于了解空气中的湿度变化推测雨量大小；在农学方面记载了用嫁接法改良果树品种等内容。这些足以说明《本草纲目》在自然科学的许多学科中都做出了重要贡献，丰富了世界科学宝库。

The compendium is not merely confined to the detailed record of pharmacology and correct narration about physiology, pathology, symptoms of diseases as well as sanitation prevention, but also covers extensive discussion on topics such as botany, zoology, mineralogy, physics, chemistry, agronomy, astronomy and meteorology, etc. For example, the book gives the description of ostrich in zoology, origin and nature of petroleum in mineralogy, and records speculating rainfall by knowing air humidity changes in physiology and improving variety of orchard through grafting in agronomy. All of these serve to show that the book has made a great contribution to many disciplines among natural sciences, enriching the world's science treasure.

(5) 辑录保存了大量古代文献

(5) Compiling and storing large amounts of ancient documents

《本草纲目》引载了16世

The book quotes and records large amounts of ancient

纪以前的大量文献资料，其中既有医药方面的，包括历代诸家本草与医药著述；也有非医药方面的，包括经史百家著述。在这许多引载的文献资料中，有的原书后来佚失，但由于《本草纲目》的摘录记载和注明了原出处，因此使某些佚失的书的部分资料得以保存下来。

literature on medicine and non-medicine before 16th century, respectively including works on materia medica and medicine written by various scholars in the past dynasties, and writings by numerous schools of thinkers. Many of those source literatures quoted in the book are lost, but some materials of them are saved because all excerpts in the book give clear record and indication about their original sources.

三 学术价值

《本草纲目》集明朝以前的药物学研究之大成，是药学史上的里程碑，总结并收载了大量新药，开辟了本草学发展的新阶段，也是我国古代文化科学宝库中的一份珍贵遗产。《本草纲目》自1596年刊行后，屡经再版，很早就流传到朝鲜和日本，并已有拉丁、英、法、德、日、朝等20余种文字的节译本或全译本，在国际上产生了重要影响。英国博物学家、进化论奠基者达尔文在其《物种起源》等书中曾数次引用《本草纲目》的资料。不少国内外学者对《本草纲目》给予高度评价。鲁迅称此书"含有丰富的宝藏"、"实在是极可宝贵的"；曾任中国科学院院长的郭沫若为李时珍题词"医中之圣，集中国药学之大成"；当代英国科学技术史学家李约瑟称赞李时珍为"药物学界中之王子"。李时珍的名字及其业绩，将永载史册，与世长存。

3 Academic value

The book, a great grab bag of studies on materia medica before the Ming Dynasty, is a landmark in the history of pharmacy. It's also a precious heritage in the ancient China's cultural science treasure with conclusion and record of numerous new medicines and the initiation of new stage on the development of herbalism. Since it was published in 1596 and reprinted repeatedly, the book had been spread quickly to Korea and Japan. It has been, totally or partially, translated into more than 20 foreign languages, including Latin, English, French, German, Japanese and Korean, etc., playing an important role in international communication. Darwin, the English natural scientist and the founder of evolution theory, had quoted materials several times from the book in his many works such as *The Origin of Species*. A lot of domestic and overseas scholars spoke highly of the book. For instance, as Lu Xun stated, it was "of abundant treasure" and "extremely precious". Guo Moruo, who was president of the Chinese Academy of Sciences, wrote an inscription for Li "a sage of physicians who epitomizes Chinese pharmacy". And Joseph Needham, the British scientific and technological historian in the contemporary era, praised Li Shizhen as "a prince in the field of materia medica". Therefore, Li's name and achievements would remain in history forever.

33 针灸大成(Zhenjiu Dacheng)

Compendium of Acupuncture and Moxibustion

一 书籍简介

《针灸大成》一书是由杨继洲(公元 1522 年—1619 年)编撰。作者出身于世医家庭,从青年时期起学习医学,对针灸学尤其钻研。他对 16 世纪以前的针灸文献进行编辑及注解,并在家传《卫生针灸玄机秘要》的基础上,结合自己的心得经验,附以自己的针灸治疗病案,于 1601 年编著成《针灸大成》。此书在《四库全书总目》中名为《针灸大全》。书内论述了经络、穴位、针灸手法与适应证等,介绍了应用针灸与药物综合治疗经验,并且还记录有针灸治疗成功与无效的病案。本书较系统地总结了明朝以前的针灸学成就经验,其中有的原书后来已经散佚,幸此书得以保存了部分资料,因而有较高的研究和应用价值,是一部在针灸界影响极大的著作。

1 A brief introduction to the book

Compendium of Acupuncture and Moxibustion (*Zhenjiu Dacheng*) was compiled by Yang Jizhou (1522—1619 A. D.), who was born in a family that had practiced medicine for generations. He learned medicine in his youth, especially working hard on the acupuncture and moxibustion. On the basis of *Mystic Secrets of Health Acupuncture* passed down in his family, he edited and annotated the documents in acupuncture and moxibustion before 16th century, and completed the book in 1601 with his learning experience and clinical case records titled *Complete Collection of Acupuncture and Moxibustion* in *Catalog of the Complete Collection of the Four Treasures* (*Siku Quanshu Zongmu*). The book elaborates meridians and collaterals, acupoints, acupuncture and moxibustion manipulations and indications, introducing integrating treating experience by applying acupuncture and moxibustion with medicine, and recording medical cases with successful and failed treating by acupuncture and moxibustion. It sums up achievements systematically in this aspect before the Ming Dynasty, among which, some original texts had been lost later and only part was preserved fortunately. So, it is of higher value of research and application and of great influence in the acupuncture and moxibustion field.

二 主要内容

全书分10卷。卷1节录《内经》、《难经》等古医籍中有关针灸的部分原文，附有杨继洲的注解；卷2—3摘引《医经小学》、《针灸聚英》、《标幽赋》、《金针赋》、《神应经》等二十余种医籍中的部分针灸歌赋，也附有杨继洲所加的注解；卷4叙述了取穴法、针具、各种针刺法等；卷5为十二经井穴、子午流注法等；卷6—卷7记述了经络、十二经穴位及主治；卷8为临床各科病症的针灸治法；卷9包括"治症总要"、名医治法、取穴法、灸治法以及杨继洲个人的针灸治疗医案等；卷10主要介绍小儿的针灸按摩治法，特别是转载的《陈氏小儿按摩经》，是很宝贵的古代小儿按摩专著，除本书外未有传本，这是现存最古老的有关按摩的文献。

《针灸大成》的主要成就与特点为：

2 The main content

The book is divided into 10 volumes. Volume 1 is the partial original text about acupuncture and moxibustion excerpted from the classic medical books, such as *Internal Classic* and *Classic of Difficulties* with annotations attached by Yang Jizhou. Volumes 2—3 quote many verses of acu-moxibustion from over 20 kinds of medical books, also with annotations attached by Yang Jizhou, for instance, *Beginner Books on Medical Classics* (*Yijing Xiaoxue*), *A Collection of Gems in Acupuncture and Moxibustion* (*Zhenjiu Juying*), *Ode to Reveal the Mysteries in Acupuncture* (*Biaoyou Fu*), *Ode to Acupuncture Needle* (*Jinzhen Fu*), and *Classic on Acupuncture Points* (*Shenying Jing*). Acupoint selection methods, needling instruments and different needling methods are introduced in volume 4. Well points of twelve meridians and midnight-noon ebb-flow acupuncture are covered in volume 5. Volumes 6 to 7 discuss the meridians and collaterals, twelve meridian points and their indications. Volume 8 is about acu-moxibustion therapy of syndromes in all clinical branches. Volume 9 covers general principles of diseases treatment, therapeutic methods of famous doctors, principles of point selection and moxibustion therapy, as well as records of Yang's personal practice. Volume 10 mainly introduces methods of acu-moxibustion and massage for children, and the reproduced book *Chen's Pediatric Massage* (*Chenshi Xiaoer Anmo Jing*) has no other edition except for the book. Thus, it's the oldest extant literature on massage and a precious monograph on pediatric massage in ancient times.

The main achievements and characteristics of *Compendium of Acupuncture and Moxibustion* are summarized as follows:

(1) 主张针灸和药物配合运用

作者没有偏于倾向针灸治疗方法，认为应该灵活地根据病情需要采取合适的治

(1) Advocating combined application of acu-moxibustion and medicines

The author holds an impartial view on the acu-moxibustion therapy, believing that suitable methods should be taken flexibly according to patients' conditions, so that

疗方法以取得最好的疗效。如文中所说"其致病也,既有不同,而其治之,亦不容一律,故药与针灸不可缺一者也";进而还指出由于疾病的部位和性质不同,治疗的方法也应有所选择:"然而疾在肠胃,非药饵不能以济;在血脉非针刺不能以及;在腠理,非熨焫不能以达;是针灸药者,医家之不可缺一者也"。作者也在书中批评了有的医家只着眼于药物治疗而忽视针灸的错误现象:"夫何诸家之术惟以药,而于针灸则并而弃之,斯何以保其元气,以收圣人寿民之仁心哉"。在《针灸大成》所载的杨继洲医案中,既有单用针灸治疗方法的,也有将针灸与药物结合应用治疗的案例。

the best curative effect can be achieved. For example, the book says "as the etiologies of diseases are different, the therapeutic methods should not be the same. Therefore, both the medicines and acu-moxibustion are indispensable in the treatment". Furthermore, it is pointed out that treating methods should also be selected according to different locations and properties of diseases: "if the disease locates in the intestines and stomach, only the medicines can relieve it; if in the blood vessels, only needling can reach it; if in the striae, only hot medicated compress and moxibustion can relieve it; acu-moxibustion and medicines are both indispensable in treatment for doctors". The author also criticizes the mistakes that some physicians just focus on medication treatment despite of acu-moxibustion, "Why some physicians simply treat patients with medicines while abandon acupuncture and moxibustion? Then how could they preserve primordial qi so that the benevolence of sages and masses who live a long life can be submitted to them?" Among Yang's practices, usage of acu-moxibustion therapy only and combined application of acu-moxibustion and medicines are all concluded in the book.

（2）指明针灸的治疗优越性

在临症治疗中杨继洲虽然主张药物与针灸配合应用,但一般而言,他认为针灸治疗有其优越性。他在引载《通玄指要赋》的"必欲治病,莫如用针"一句话时,解释说:"夫治病之法,有药饵,然药饵或出于幽远之方,有时缺少,而又有新陈之不等,真伪之不同,其何以奏肤功、起沉疴也? 惟精于针,可以随身带用,以备缓急。"他对《标幽赋》的"拯

（2）Indicating the superiority of acu-moxibustion in treatment

Yang Jizhou advocates the combined application of medicines with acu-moxibustion in clinical treatment, but generally speaking, what he emphasizes is the superiority of acu-moxibustion therapy. As to the sentence "it would be better to use needles for diseases treatment" he quotes from *Ode of the Essentials for Penetrating Mysteries* (*Tongxuan Zhiyao Fu*), he explains that medicine is necessary for treatment, however, some are grown afar and in shortage sometimes, while others are different, being old or fresh, genuine or fake. Therefore, how can they get the curative effect? Only needling treatment is convenient in case of emergency. He emphasizes on the advantages of acu-moxibustion again when annotating "needle is a magic

救之法，妙用者针”这句话进行注解时，再次强调针灸的有利特点，说：“劫病之功，莫捷于针灸。故《素问》诸书，为之首载，缓、和、扁、华，俱以此称神医。盖一针中穴，病者应手而起，诚医家之所先也。……又语云：一针、二灸、三服药。则针灸为妙用可知。业医者奈之何不亟讲乎？”

saving method" from *Ode to Reveal the Mysteries in Acupuncture*. He says "the success of curing diseases only owe to acu-moxibustion therapy. Therefore, it was first-recorded in books such as *Plain Questions*. Yi Huan, Yi He, Bian Que and Hua Tuo were called highly-skilled doctors for their needling. Needling a certain point can make patient recover instantly, and so physicians should choose acupuncture first." He also says that "giving priority to acupuncture, then moxibustion and taking medicines at last, thus the effect of acupuncture can be clearly seen. But why don't doctors take this therapy as soon as possible?"

(3) 发展“透穴针治法”

杨继洲在元代王国瑞的《扁鹊神应针灸玉龙经》对偏头痛一针两穴治法基础上，发展了多种透穴针治法。如他所记载的治疗偏头痛疾病，可以使用针刺方法，选取丝竹空穴位针刺后，沿皮肤浅层向后透率谷穴位，一针两穴的透穴方法具有很好的治疗头痛效果。其他又记载了针刺风池穴位一寸半后横向透刺风府穴可以治疗头痛疾病，采用针刺膝关穴横针透膝眼治疗两腿疼痛膝部红肿者，采用针刺液门穴沿皮向后透阳池穴治疗手臂红肿连腕疼痛者，为后世的透穴治疗提供了丰富经验。

(3) Developing "point-through-point acupuncture method"

On the basis of "one needle, two points" method for migraine in *Bian Que Responding to Jade Dragon Verses on Acu-moxibustion* (*Bianque Shenying Zhenjiu Yulong Jing*) written by Wang Guorui in the Yuan Dynasty, Yang Jizhou develops many kinds of point through point acupuncture treatment. For example, the method recorded for treating migraine is acupuncture therapy. Selecting and puncturing on Sizhukong (TE 23) first, then inserting backwards along the superficial layer of skin to Shuaigu point (GB 8), and this point through point acupuncture has a good treating effect on headache. Among others, there is another record of curing headache by puncturing Fengchi (GB 20) 1.5 *cun* and then penetrating Fengfu (GV 16) laterally. There are also records of treating leg pain and redness of knees through puncturing Xiguan joint (LR 7) and then penetrating Xiyan (EX-LE 5) laterally. Treating redness and swelling of arms and waist pain by puncturing Yemen (TE 2) first and then inserting backwards along the skin to penetrate Yangchi (TE 4). All of which provide rich experience in point-through-point acupuncture method for the later generations.

(4) 创造发展了多种针刺手法

在针刺手法方面，杨继洲阐明了持针、进针、退针、搓针、捻针、留针及摇针等手法要点，并编写成简明易记的"十二字歌"以有利于学习者掌握。此外《针灸大成》还记载介绍了烧山火、透天凉、苍龙摆尾、赤凤摇头、龙虎交战、龙虎升降、子午补泻等多种针刺手法。

(4) Creating and developing many acupuncture manipulations

On the acupuncture manipulations, many key points of needling are elaborated in the book, such as holding, inserting, withdrawing, twisting, twirling, rotating, retaining, shaking and so on. Yang Jizhou compiles these manipulations into "Songs of 12 words", which makes those points brief and easy for learners to grasp. Besides, the book also records varieties of acupuncture manipulations, such as setting the mountain on fire (*Shao Shan Huo*), heaven-penetrating cooling (*Tou Tian Liang*), dragon wagging its tail (*Cang Long Bai Wei*), red phoenix shaking its head (*Chi Feng Yao Tou*), dragon-tiger contending (*Long Hu Jiao Zhan*), lifting and descending of dragon and tiger (*Long Hu Sheng Jiang*) and midnight-noon reinforcement and reduction (*Zi Wu Bu Xie*), etc.

(5) 提出灸法的相关使用原则

《针灸大成》中对头部提出不宜多灸的原则。古代施行灸术，往往数十壮甚至百壮以上，而头部为诸阳之会，肌肉单薄，确不宜多灸，即使现今灸治的壮数已大为减少，但"头不可多灸"的观点，仍然是值得重视的。书中还阐明了掌握灸治壮数的原则，作者认为灸也需要注意所灸的壮数，因为要考虑每个人的个体差异，人体的机体皮肤肌肉特点不同，有厚薄、深浅的不同，所以不可一概而论，需要根据患者的机体特点而加以灵活变化，不可以拘泥于固定的数目，并且举出少商、承浆、少冲、涌泉等穴位灸量不宜太

(5) Proposing relevant principles for applying moxibustion therapy

In *Compendium of Acupuncture and Moxibustion*, it is advised that doctors should take less moxibustion treatment on the head. There were often tens or hundreds of moxas in the past, however, the head should not take more moxibustion as it is the convergence of yang with thin muscle. It is still worth attention nowadays even the number of cones is greatly reduced. The book also introduces the principles of adjusting cone number in moxibustion therapy, taking into consideration of all individual differences, including characteristics, thickness and depth of skin and muscle, etc. The author holds that number of cones should be flexibly adjusted, instead of sticking to the fixed number. The author also recommends that dosage of moxibustion should be moderate on acupoints like Shaoshang (LU 11), Chengjiang (CV 24), Shaochong (HT 9) and Yongquan (KI 1), otherwise it would be harmful. Better curative effect can be available only with more dosage of moxibustion on

大,过则有害;章门、膏肓、曲池、足三里等穴位灸量可大些才能取得较好的疗效。

the acupoints like Zhangmen (LR 13), Gaohuang (BL 43), Quchi (LI 11) and Zusanli (ST 36).

三 学术价值

总之,《针灸大成》是一部内容相当丰富的针灸专书,该书广收前人针灸著述,使某些针灸资料得以流传后世,在针灸学发展史上起到了承前启后的重要作用,并且很早就流传到日本等国,在国内外都有相当的影响。至今各种版本已达50余种,并被翻译成德、法、英、日等国文字,受到世界许多国家医学界的重视。

3 Academic value

In short, *Compendium of Acupuncture and Moxibustion* is a monograph on acu-moxibustion with rich content. It widely integrates writings of former people, making some materials on acu-moxibustion handed down in the later generations. It plays an important role in inheriting the past and ushering in the future in the history of acu-moxibustion. Being spread to Japan and other countries very early, it has great influence at home and abroad. So far, it has more than 50 versions, which have been translated into German, French, English and Japanese, etc., receiving great attention in the medical fields of many countries.

34 外科正宗(Waike Zhengzong)

Orthodox Manual of External Medicine

一 书籍简介

《外科正宗》是由明朝的著名外科学家陈实功(公元1555年—1636年)所著,他在外科方面钻研40余年,为了使外科医学能够让更多的人重视起来,让更多的行医者掌握方法技巧,他晚年不顾身体虚弱,根据自己多年行医的丰富经验和明朝以前外科医学方面的部分成就,于公元1617年撰写了这部重要的外科医学著作《外科正宗》,集中体现了他的学术思想。书中理论讨论精辟,治法得当,并附若干医案,令人信服,得以"列症最详,论治最精"著称,反映了明朝以前我国外科学的重要成就。

1 A brief introduction to the book

Orthodox Manual of External Medicine (*Waike Zhengzong*) was compiled by Chen Shigong (1555—1636 A. D.), a famous surgeon in the Ming Dynasty. He engaged in the surgery for more than 40 years. In order to make more people pay attention to the surgical medicine and more medical practitioners grasp techniques, in spite of weak constitution in his old age, he compiled the significant surgical work in 1617 A. D. on the basis of his abundant experience of medical practice for many years and the achievements in this aspect before the Ming Dynasty. It is the concentrated embodiment of his academic idea, which convinces us with penetrating discussion on theory, appropriate treatment and numerous medical cases. Thus, the book is known for incisive discussion on treatment with detailed syndromes listed, reflecting the significant achievement in surgery before the Ming Dynasty.

二 主要内容

全书共分为4卷,包括157篇,对痈疽、疔疮、流注、瘰疬、瘿瘤、肠痈、痔疮、白癜风、烫伤、疥疮等外伤,皮肤、五官科疾病进行了分门逐类的论述,从各医家对病因的认识到临床症状和特点,以及各

2 The main content

The book is divided into 4 volumes, including 157 chapters. Classified discussions are made on trauma, skin disease and ENT (ear, nose and throat) diseases such as ulcer, boil, multiple abscess, scrofula, goiter and tumor, appendicitis, pile, leukoderma, scald, scabies, etc. The discussions range from physicians' recognition on etiology to clinical symptoms and characteristics, as well as therapeutic

种病症的治疗方法，手术的适应证、禁忌等，都做了详细的论述。该书的要点主要有：

methods for various diseases, indication and contraindication of operations. The main points of the book are as follows:

（1）内外并治，重视“消托补”的外科治疗总原则

在外科的治疗原则上，陈实功提出内外治法并重的原则。内治重视“托”与调脾胃。因为“脾胃盛，使脓秽自排、毒气自解、死肉自溃、新肉自生、饮食自进、疮口自敛”。这些“自”均反映了机体自身的恢复调节能力，也说明他充分认识到人体内在因素的作用。外治则强调“使毒外出为第一”，常用腐蚀药和刀针，清除坏死组织、切开引流以达到“开户逐贼”的效果。对脓肿治疗则强调要“开户逐贼”，“使毒外出为第一”，运用刀、针扩创引流，或采用腐蚀药清除坏死组织。同时作者提出了外科治疗的总原则“消托补”，其中消法适用于肿疡早期；托法适用于肿疡后期和溃疡早期；补法侧重于溃疡后期。陈实功认为内科疾病不一定会影响到肢体外部，但是外科疾病却是必有内在的根源。因此对于外科疾病他也很重视调理脾胃，主张通过调理脾胃，扶助正气，这样有益于脓肿的排出或者外科创口的愈合，即多采用托、补二法。

(1) Attaching importance to "resolving, expelling and reinforcing method" of surgical treatment through internal-external therapy

On the principles of surgical treatment, Chen Shigong attaches equal importance to the internal and external therapy. The former stresses on expelling and regulating spleen and stomach as sufficient spleen and stomach can make pus released, mephitis detoxified, carrion festered, new flesh developed, diet being fed and an open sore healed up all by themselves, which reflects the ability of body recovery by itself and his full recognition on the role of body's internal factors. External therapy, however, emphasizes on releasing toxicity first. Escharotica and knife-needle are often used to clear off necrotic tissues and cut off drainage to reach the effect of clearance. As for abscess treatment, he lays stress on expelling the toxicity in the first place by applying knife and needle in the drainage debridement, or utilizing escharotica to clear off necrotic tissues. Meanwhile, the author proposes overall principle of "resolving, expelling and reinforcing method" in the surgical treatment. Among which, resolving method is applicable for tumor in the early stage, expelling method is for tumor in the later stage and ulcer in the early stage, and reinforcing method is mainly for ulcer in the later stage. Chen Shigong believes that diseases of internal department may not affect the outer parts of limbs, but there must be inner root for surgical diseases. Therefore, he also attaches importance to spleen and stomach regulation, advocating to support healthy qi by regulating the function of spleen and stomach, which is beneficial for the discharge of abscess and healing of surgical wound.

(2) 对癌肿有深刻的认识

作者在当时已经对癌肿类疾病有深刻的认识,观察到癌肿属于不治之症状,只能延长生命,并指出他所创的“和荣散坚丸”、“阿魏化坚膏”等仅仅是“缓命药也”。他认为肿瘤只有及早发现,才能摸清病源,以便能够及早治疗,或许尚有一线希望治愈。此外他对癌肿进行了分类,有乳岩(乳腺癌)、翻花疮(皮肤癌)、茧唇(唇癌)、颈疮(淋巴癌)、鼻咽以及内脏等癌肿,把癌肿命名为“失荣”。在论述病因时,他指出忧郁、心愿不遂以及不良刺激等因素是重要原因。他的这些见解提高了中医对癌肿的认识,一些论述至今还有科学价值。

(2) Understanding cancerous swelling profoundly

At that time, the author already had profound recognition for diseases of cancerous swelling. He observes that patients with the syndrome can not be cured but only be survived by prolonging the lifespan. It is pointed out that some medicines he creates are simply to delay the dying date, such as Relieving Swelling and Dissipating Hardness Pill and Awei Hardness-dissolving Paste. He believes that only by finding tumor earlier, can the more possibilities we have to explore the causes and to cure the disease. Besides, he categorizes the cancerous swelling, including mammary carcinoma (breast cancer), luxuriant granulation (skin cancer), cocoon lips (lip cancer), neck sore (lymphoma), nasopharynx and viscera cancer. On the discussion of etiology, depression, aspiration without being realized and pessimal stimulation are all categorized as the important reasons for the disease. With his views, TCM's recognition on cancerous swelling has been improved, and some of his discussion are of scientific value till now.

(3) 提高了很多外科手术水平

作者非常善于设计制造许多简单而有效的器械,提高了各种外科手术的水平。书中记载有鼻息肉摘除术、咽喉食道铁针取出术、截肢术、挂线治瘘疗法等多种外科治疗手术。如记载治疗误吞针铁、骨刺鲠于咽部,用一个像龙眼大小的麻线团,系上丝线,用温水淋湿,让患者急速吞下,然后扯住留在外面的丝线,徐徐拉出,针、铁、骨刺就会入麻团而被扯出。如骨刺难以扯出,就用“乌龙针法推之”,即

(3) Promoting the level of various surgical operations

The author is very good at manufacturing simple and effective medical devices, promoting the level of various surgical operations. Many surgical operations are recorded in the book, such as polypectomy, pulling steel needle out from throat and esophagus, amputation, seton for fistula treatment. For example, if steel needle is mistakenly swallowed and fishbone is stuck in one's throat, let the patient rapidly swallow a ball of twine attached to silk thread and wetted with warm water. After being swallowed by patients, then grasp the silk thread left outside and pull it out slowly. Afterwards, needle, steel and fishbone would be stuck in the twine and dragged out. If it is difficult to pull fishbone out, "oolong needle method" would be applied: burning iron wire to be soft, wrapping it with longan-sized beeswax and winding up a silk thread outside,

用烧软的铁线,裹上龙眼大的黄蜡,外用丝线缠好,推入咽喉内鲠骨之处,骨刺就会顺着被推到胃部。又如摘除鼻痔,用细钢箸两根,箸端各钻一孔用丝线穿孔,彼此相距几分,使用时,将箸头伸入鼻内痔根上,然后将管线绞紧,向下一拔,痔就应手而落。此外,作者在截肢、气管缝合、落耳再植、下颌骨脱臼复位等大小外科手术,以及对痔瘘采用枯痔散、枯痔钉、护痔膏、挂线等外治疗法上,都有不同程度的发现和提高。其中对下颏骨脱臼的治疗整复手术,完全符合现代医学的要求,直到现在仍一直沿用。

then pushing it to where the fishbone exists in the throat, which would drop along the stomach. Another case is removing rhinopolypus with two fine steel chopsticks drilled with a hole respectively, and punching holes with a silk thread several centimeters apart. Dipping the end of the chopsticks into the root of rhinopolypus when using them, then have the thread taut and pluck it downwards, the rhinopolypus would then fall down. Besides, the author also has different degrees of discovery and improvement in various surgical operations, as well as external therapies, such as amputation, bronchial suture, ear replantation, dislocation and reduction of mandible and some therapies utilized in anal fistula, for instance, alum hemorrhoid-desiccating powder and nails, hemorrhoid ointment, and seton. Among which, the treating and reduction operation on the dislocation of mandible, totally conform with the command of modern medicine and is still in use today.

三 学术价值

《外科正宗》的研究和探索十分珍贵,对现代临床治疗都有一定的启示。全书综述了自唐朝以来历代外科中有效治疗经验,科学性强,论述精辟,能充分代表明代时期我国外科医学的巨大成就,具有较高的学习研究价值。《外科正宗》印行后也广为流传,并流传到日本等国,成为中医外科的经典著作。

3 Academic value

With precious research and exploration, *Orthodox Manual of External Medicine* has a certain inspiration for modern clinical treatment. It has summed up effective treating experience in the surgical department of past dynasties since the Tang Dynasty. With scientific content and penetrating elaboration, the book can fully represent great achievements in the surgical medicine of the Ming Dynasty, so it is of higher value for study and research. After being published, *Orthodox Manual of External Medicine* has been introduced to some foreign countries like Japan. The book proves to be a classic work on the surgical department of TCM.

35 景岳全书(Jingyue Quanshu)

Jing Yue's Collected Works

一 书籍简介

《景岳全书》是明朝著名医家张介宾(公元1563年—1640年)晚年的一部力作。张介宾字景岳,自幼聪明好学,博览经史百家,其父曾先教他读《内经》,十四岁带他进京拜名医为师。壮年时他投笔从戎,遍历东北各地,后卸职回乡专攻医学,把广泛的经史、天文、术数、堪舆、律吕、兵法等知识运用到医学之中,很快成为名医,求诊者络绎不绝。他对中医内科学的贡献相当突出,其医学思想起初受朱震亨的理论影响,赞同朱氏"阳常有余,阴常不足"的论点。后来根据《内经》"阴平阳秘,精神乃治"观点而提出"阳非有余"、"真阴不足"以及"人体虚多实少"等理论。张介宾非常重视《内经》,对《素问》和《灵枢》进行了30多年研究,注重在实践中检验和发展医学理论,晚年结合个人丰富的临症经验和独到的

1 A brief introduction to the book

Jing Yue's Collected Works (*Jingyue Quanshu*) is a masterpiece of Zhang Jiebin (1563—1640 A. D.), a famous physician in the Ming Dynasty, which was compiled in his old age. Zhang Jiebin, whose courtesy name is Jing Yue, was intelligent and fond of study when he was young. He read widely about classics, histories and different schools of thought. His father had taught him how to read *Internal Classic* and then took him to learn from famous doctors in Beijing. He gave up civilian pursuits to join the army in his middle age, traveling around all places of the north-eastern China. Later, he specialized in medicine as he was relieved of his position and back to hometown. Soon, he became a prominent doctor by applying extensive knowledge, including classics and histories, astronomy, divination, geomancy, temperament and art of war, to medicine. People seeking medical consultation came to see him in an endless stream. He made salient contributions to the internal medicine of TCM. In the first place, his medical thought was influenced by the theory of Zhu Zhenheng, whose argument that "yang being often in excess while yin being often deficient" was in line with his own idea. Later, he proposed that "yang isn't always surplus", "true yin is insufficient" and "deficiency is more than excess in human body" according to the idea in *Internal Classic* that "Only when yin is at peace and yang is compact can essence-spirit be normal." Zhang Jingyue attached great attention to *Internal Classic*. He worked on

理论，于1624年撰成《景岳全书》一书，这是一部较完整的记载临床各科理法方药的书籍。

Plain Questions and *Miraculous Pivot* for more than 30 years, paying more attention to examine and develop medical theory in the practice. Combining with his abundant clinical experience and original theory, Zhang completed the book in 1624, which completely recorded the principle-method-recipe-medicines in different clinical branches.

二 主要内容

该书共分24集，包括64卷。内容涉及中医基础理论、诊断治法、内外妇儿临床各科、治法方剂、本草药性等内容囊括无遗，全面而精详。其主要的思想为：

2 The main content

The book is divided into 24 collections, including 64 volumes. It is comprehensive and detailed in content, covering basic theory of TCM, diagnosis and treatment, clinical departments (department of internal medicine, surgery, gynecology and pediatrics), therapeutic methods and herbal properties. The main ideas are characterized as follows:

(1) 重视元阴、元阳对人体的重要性

张介宾在他书籍中反复论述了元阴、元阳对人体的重要性，并且把两者归根于命门的水火，认为元阴元阳是造化之源泉，性命之根本。他认为阳气是人体阴阳矛盾中的主导方面，原因是万物之生由乎阳，万物之死亦由乎阳。人之生长壮老，皆由阳气为之主，精血津液之生成，皆由阳气为之化。基于阳气为主导的思想而指出“阳强则寿，阳衰则夭”，从而提出阳气的盛衰关系着人之寿夭的论点。同时他也指出生命之所依赖者是形体，“形”赖精血以养，精血是产生形体和维持形体不衰的物质基础。“凡欲治病者，必以形体为主；欲治形者，必

(1) Paying attention to the importance of primordial yin and yang to human body

In his book, Zhang Jiebin discusses the importance of primordial yin and yang to human body. He attributes them to the fire and water of the vital gate (GV 4), believing that they are the sources of nature, the basic point of life. As both the creation and death of all things are from yang, he holds yang qi plays dominant role in the yin-yang contradiction of human body. The growth, constitution and lifespan are all governed by the yang qi and the production of essence, blood and body fluid is transformed by yang qi. Therefore, based on the theory that yang qi playing a leading role, he points out that strong yang may cause longevity, otherwise resulting in earlier death. Furthermore, he puts forward that the ebb and flow of yang qi pertain to the lifespan of human beings. Meanwhile, he proposes that body is what the life depends on. “Shape” is nurtured by essence and blood, which is the material base to create body and maintain its appearance. “People who desire to get recovered from diseases must be mainly treated with physique. Others who want to cure physique must be treated

以精血为先”、“今人之病阴虚者十常八九”。张介宾在这方面的详尽论述,是对医学理论的推进与深化。他力主补益元阴和元阳,强调在进行补阴时适当选用补阳药,补阳时适当选用补阴药,指出“此又阴阳相济之妙用也”,并且认为“善补阳者必于阴中求阳,则阳得阴助而生化无穷;善补阴者必于阳中求阴,则阴得阳升而泉源不竭。”他所创制的左归丸旨在壮水之主,以培元阴而精血自充。在培补精血的方剂中皆重用熟地、山茱萸、枸杞、山药、菟丝子、当归、人参等药。这些药物一般都有补益精血、滋养真阴、培固本元的作用,对于年老体虚之人,尤其适宜。

with essence and blood”; “there are nine out of ten patients whose yin are in deficiency”. In this aspect, the detailed explanation given by Zhang Jiebin is proved to be the advancement and deepening of the medical theory. He strongly advocates tonifying primordial yin and yang, emphasizing on properly selecting yang tonics when nourishing yin and vice versa. He points out that “it is a wonderful method to get yin and yang coordinated each other”. He also thinks that “people who are good at tonifying yang should get it from yin, then transformation of yang would be endless, and vice versa.” He created Left-Restoring Pill(Zuogui Wan) to cultivate primordial yin, so that essence and blood would be sufficient in itself. Some medicines are mainly used in prescriptions tonifying essence and blood, such as prepared rehmannia root (shudihuang), asiatic cornelian cherry fruit (shanzhuyu), barbary wolfberry fruit (gouqi), common yam rhizome (shanyao), dodder seed (tusizi), Chinese angelica, ginseng, etc. As for the function of the nourishment of essence, blood, and true yin, as well as the reinforcement of original vitality, these drugs are particular suitable for the weak and old people.

(2) 探索人之寿夭的影响因素

张介宾对人之寿夭的问题进行了积极的研究和探索,提出了自己卓有成效的见识。他认为:“先天强厚者多寿,先天薄弱者多夭;后天培养者寿者更寿,后天所削者夭者更夭”,认识到人的寿命长短与先天因素和身体的禀赋有关系,但是也可以通过后天的培养而改变,从而说明了人之寿夭在很大程度上取决于人之本身是否注意摄养。即先天

(2) Exploring the factors influencing the lifespan of people

Zhang Jiebin makes active research and exploration on the question of human's lifespan, proposing a highly effective view. He thinks that “the better inborn constitution he/she has and the more cultivation of his/her body, the longer he/she lives, and vice versa”. He recognizes that the lifespan is related to instinctive factors and natural endowment, which can be changed, however, through cultivation acquired later in one's life. Therefore, to a great extent, it depends on whether people themselves pay attention to conserving health or not. It means, on one

强者寿,先天弱者夭;后天培养者寿,后天失养者夭;先天强者,后天又慎之以养,则寿者更寿;先天弱者,后天又失之以养,则夭者更夭。这种观点反映了张介宾认识到人的主观能动性在抗老延年中起着积极作用。这对于加强后天培养,提高人类寿命具有重要的指导意义。

hand, people with good inborn constitution would live a longer life if they cultivate themselves better, otherwise they would die early without nourishment; on the other hand, people with poor original physique would live a shorter life if they don't take care of nourishing themselves. The opinion reflects that Zhang Jiebin has recognized that subjective initiative plays a positive role in anti-aging and prolonging life. It is of significant guidance to reinforce nurture and raise longevity of human beings.

(3) 重视形体与心理之间的关系

张介宾从临床经验中提出了对形体和心理之间关系的一系列精辟的见解,如神明元气论、神形统一论和个性先天禀赋论。他认为精神从本质上说是元气,元气充沛则精神昌盛。他反对心身二元论,主张形神统一说,神离不开形,神是形的作用,"神自形生",神支配着形,失去了神,形就丧失了存在的意义。在七情损伤与疾病的关系上他认为存在双向性影响,七情损伤可以致病,疾病也会导致七情损伤。这些分析身心关系复杂性的观点,为分析精神因素变化的实质奠定了方法论基础。在这一思想指导下,他非常重视心理治疗的作用及心理健康在预防中的作用。强调养神是预防疾病的首要环节,在具体的养神方法上,主张要善于自我调节,行动适度不可使之过,不可放纵情欲。

(3) Paying attention to the relations between body and psychology

Zhang Jiebin puts forward a series of profound insights on the relations between body and psychology, for instance, discussion on vitality of spirit mind, unity of shape and mind, and natural endowment of personality. He believes that spirit is vitality by nature. With vigorous primordial qi, it would be full of spirit and energy. He opposes dualism on mind and body and advocates unity of them. The mind, which cannot be separate from the body, is the function of the body. The shape would lose its existing meaning without the dominance of mind. On the relations between injury of seven emotions and diseases, he believes there exists two-way influence, the former could cause the latter and vice versa. These views on the complexity of body-mind relations lay methodological foundations for the analysis on the changing essence of spiritual factors. Under the guidance, he attaches great attention to the role of psychological treatment and mental health in prevention. Mind nourishment is emphasized to be the first step for the prevention of diseases. As for the specific method, he advocates self-regulation with moderate action and passion.

三 学术价值

《景岳全书》中所反映的作者的理论与所创方剂，对后世产生了较大的影响。这部书是记录了张介宾毕生治病经验和中医学术成果的综合性著作。书中首创"补、和、攻、散、寒、热、固、因"的方药八阵分类新法，反映了其一生临床心得、处方体会与用药特长的融合。

3 Academic value

The theory and prescriptions the author shows in *Jing Yue's Collected Works* bring greater influence to the later generations. It is an integrated work recording academic achievements of TCM and treatment experience throughout Zhang Jiebin's life. The initiative classification method in this book, "eight arrays of formulas" (supplementing, harmonizing, offensive, dissipating, cold, heat, securing and adaptation), reflects the integration of his clinical understanding, recipe experience and medication specialty.

36 瘟疫论(Wenyi Lun)

Treatise on Pestilence

一 书籍简介

《瘟疫论》,又称《温疫论》,是中国第一部系统研究急性传染病的医学书籍。作者是在中医学史上创立温病学说中做出杰出贡献的著名医家吴有性。我国在医学文献中所记载的古代发生的传染病不断,曾经多次造成大批人员死亡。我国历代医家对传染病的防治都十分重视,如《黄帝内经》、《伤寒论》、《诸病源候论》等著名医著中都有防治传染病经验的记载,但这些记载都不系统。《瘟疫论》一书提出对传染病病因的认识不同于以往的"六气学说",而是感天地之疫气致病。《瘟疫论》将瘟疫与其他热性病区别开来,从而使传染病病因突破了前人六气学说的束缚,在我国第一次建立了以机体抗病功能不良、感染戾气为发病原因的新论点。作者吴有性,字又可,毕生以医为业,其所生活的时代正是传染病大流行的时候。当时大疫不断,吴有性亲身经历了公元 1641 年

1 A brief introduction to the book

Treatise on Pestilence (*Wenyi Lun*), is the first medical book researching on the acute infectious diseases systematically. The author Wu Youxing was one of the famous physicians who made excellent contributions to the creation of theory of warm diseases in the TCM history. As the infectious diseases happened in ancient times were recorded constantly in the medical books, triggering a large number of casualties for many times, therefore, the treatment and prevention of infectious diseases were attached great attention by physicians through the ages in China. Though there are records of treating experience in many famous medical books such as *Huangdi's Internal Classic*, *Treatise on Cold Damage* , *Treatise on Causes and Manifestations of Various Diseases*, these records are unsystematic. *Treatise on Pestilence* puts forward that the etiology of infectious diseases is different from former "six-qi theory", instead, it is caused by exogenous pathogenic factors. The book differentiates plague diseases from other febrile diseases, breaking through the views on etiology held by former people and establishing a new argument that poor body functions of disease resistance resulting in pestilent qi. The author Wu Youxing, who styled himself as You Ke, worked on medicine throughout his life. Precisely, the epidemic disease was prevalent in the time he lived in. At that

流行在河北、山东、江苏、浙江等省的瘟疫(传染病)。他通过亲身观察和诊病施药的大量实践,在继承前人有关温病论述材料的基础上,结合自己的实践经验,创造性地提出了温病不同于伤寒的系统见解,于1642年编著《瘟疫论》,为温病学说创立起到了奠基作用。

time, heavy pestilences constantly happened. Wu Youxing experienced the plague diseases popular in Hebei, Shandong, Jiangsu and Zhejiang. Based on the former expounding materials on plague diseases with his own practical experience, he proposed systematic views that warm disease was different from typhoid fever by observation on his own and a lot of practice through diagnosis and medication. *Treatise on Pestilence* was compiled in 1642, laying a foundation for the establishment of theory of warm diseases.

二 主要内容

《瘟疫论》分为2卷,上卷载论文50篇,阐述瘟疫之病因、病机、证候、治疗,并从多方面论述瘟疫与伤寒的不同。下卷载文36篇,着重论述瘟疫的兼证和诊治。该书在传染病医学理论方面具有重要的贡献价值。

2 The main content

Treatise on Pestilence is divided into 2 volumes. Volume 1 contains 50 essays, expounding the etiology, pathogenesis, syndromes and treatment of pestilence, as well as differences between warm disease and typhoid fever from many aspects. There are 36 essays in volume 2, emphasizing on the accompanied symptoms and diagnosis and treatment of pestilence. The book embraces significant value of contribution in the medical theory of infectious diseases.

(1) 提出传染病的病因观—“戾气学说”

《瘟疫论》原序说:“瘟疫之为病,非风、非寒、非暑、非湿,乃天地之间别有一种异气所感。”作者在书中又称这种异气为杂气、戾气、疫气等,他就瘟疫病的致病原因,提出了“戾气学说”这一伟大创见,突破了明朝以前的医家对疫病病因所持的时气说、伏气说、瘴气说以及百病皆生于六气的论点,脱离了前人学说的旧窠。而是否致病,既与戾气的量、毒力大小有关,也与人体

(1) Proposing the etiology of infectious diseases—“the theory of epidemic pathogen”

Preface in the book writes: “the reason why pestilence is a disease is that it is an abnormal qi among the heaven and earth, instead of wind, cold, heat or humidity”. The author also calls it miscellaneous qi, epidemic pathogen and pestilent qi. As for the pathogenic factors of pestilence, overcoming the traditional theories, he proposes the great and innovative opinion——“ the theory of epidemic pathogen”, making a breakthrough in those arguments held by physicians before the Ming Dynasty, such as seasonal epidemic pathogen, latent qi and miasmic qi, as well as all diseases originating from six qi. Pathogenic factors, however, are related to the volume of epidemic pathogen,

抵抗力强弱有关。

power of toxicity and strength of body resistance.

（2）指出了传染病的主要传染途径

作者认为在传染病发病过程中，病因"戾气"常常通过口鼻侵犯人体，使人感染瘟疫，科学地预见了传染病的主要传染途径是从"口鼻而入"，突破了前人关于"外邪伤人皆从皮毛而入"的笼统观点。同时说明了人体感染戾气的方式"有天受，有传染，所感虽殊，其病则一。"所谓"天受"是指通过自然界空气传播，"传染"则是指通过患者接触传播。但是，只要是同一种戾气，不论是"天受"或是"传染"，所引起的疫病则是相同的。

(2) Pointing out the main routes of infection

The author believes that "epidemic pathogen" often invades body and makes people infected during the infectious diseases attack through mouth and nose. It scientifically foresees the main routes of infectious diseases are "from nose and mouth", breaking through the previous general view of "evil pathogens invade body from the skin only". Though the routes are different, from airborne transmission or from people to people, the pathogenic factors are the same. The so-called "airborne transmission" refers to transfer via air while "from people to people" means contact transmission by patients. As long as it is the same epidemic pathogen, however, the pestilence is alike no matter that is from the air or from people.

（3）指出了传染病的病原致病特异性

作者在书中描述了瘟疫有强烈的传染性，"无问老幼，触者皆病"，但同时也指出虽然人和畜禽都会因戾气致病，但是戾气的种类不同，所引起的疾病也就不同；而且人类的疫病和禽兽的瘟疫是由不同的戾气所引起的。"然牛病而羊不病，鸡病而鸭不病，人病而禽兽不病，究其所伤不同，因其气各异也。"这个"异"字反映出对病原致病的特异性的认识。另外在发病症状上，作者也指出因为戾气的种类不同，所引起的疾病也不同，

(3) Indicating specificity on pathogens of infectious diseases

The author describes the strong infectiousness of pestilence, "all people infected would be sick no matter old or young". Meanwhile, it indicates that people and livestock can get infected because of epidemic pathogen, but different epidemic pathogens lead to different diseases. Furthermore, pestilence of human beings and livestock is caused by different epidemic pathogens. "Cows are sick, but sheep are not; chickens are ill, but ducks are not; so are people and livestock. Exactly, it is because of the different qi with the varied illness". The word "different" has reflected the recognition of specificity on pathogens. Besides, as for disease symptoms, the author also indicates that the affected parts of zang organs are varied because of various kinds of epidemic pathogen, so did the incurred diseases. "Some qi specially goes to certain zang-fu viscera

侵犯的脏器部位也不一,"适有某气专入某脏腑经络,专发为某病。"反映出病原致病症状表现方面的特异性。

and meridians and collaterals, causing specific diseases", which shows the specificity on symptom appearance of different pathogens.

(4) 正确地阐明了戾气、人体、疾病三者之间的关系

《瘟疫论》中指出当人体感受戾气之后,是否致病取决于戾气的量、毒力与人体的抵抗力。如指出是否立即发病与感受邪气的深浅程度有关,"其感之深者,中而即发,感之浅者,邪不胜正,未能顿发";但是如果邪气猛烈,毒力大,无论强弱都易患病,"气来之厉,不论强弱,正气稍衰者,触之即病";同时也看到人体本身的正气充沛所具备的抵抗力,"本气充满,邪不易入,本气适逢亏欠,呼吸之间,外邪因而乘之","或遇饥饱劳碌,忧思气怒,正气被伤,邪气始得张溢。"这些都反映出戾气、人体、疾病三者之间的辨证关系。

(4) Expounding correctly the relations among epidemic pathogen, human body and diseases

Treatise on Pestilence points out that whether diseases occur depends on the volume of epidemic pathogen, power of toxicity, and resistance of human body after human body infected with epidemic pathogen. For example, "With severe infection, the disease attacks instantly, otherwise, the pathogenic qi would be defeated and fail to incur disease". If the pathogenic qi is, however, violent with powerful toxicity, people would get diseases easily. "People with weak healthy qi would be sick no matter the epidemic pathogens are severe or not". Meanwhile, the resistance can be seen from people who have vigorous healthy qi in their bodies. "Sufficient healthy qi would resist the invasion of pathogenic qi, otherwise, evil qi would get into the body during breaths", "pathogenic qi begins to spread with starvation or toil, over-thought or anger sometimes because healthy qi is hurt", which all indicates the dialectical relations among epidemic pathogens, human body and diseases.

(5) 提出了治疗疫病的基本原则和注意点

《瘟疫论》对疫病治疗提出了基本原则,即"客邪贵乎早逐","客邪"就是指侵犯人体致病的邪气,对于病邪越早祛除越好,有利于疾病的好转和痊愈。为了早日逐出疫邪,吴有性主张早用攻下法祛邪,但他同时又提出了几方面的注意

(5) Putting forward basic principles and key points for the treatment of pestilence

Treatise on Pestilence puts forward basic principles for the treatment of pestilence—"it's better to remove *Invaded Evil* as early as possible". "*Invaded Evil*" refers to pathogenic qi that infringes human body and triggers diseases. The earlier pathogenic factors are expelled, the better patients recover from diseases. Wu Youxing advocates offensive purgative method to remove the pathogenic qi. He also puts

点，如“要量人之虚实，度邪之轻重，察病之缓急，揣邪气离膜原之多寡，然后药不空投，投药无太过不及之弊。”即在用药攻邪方面，需要结合考虑患者的体质虚实，邪气的轻重，病情的缓急状况，邪气在身体内的部位深浅等因素而辨证施药，不可让药物空投而无效。

forward notes in several aspects. For example, as for treating pathogenic qi with medicines, many factors should be taken into consideration before dialectic medication, such as deficiency and excess of patients' constitutions, the degree of pathogenic qi, the urgency of disease and depth of pathogen inside the body, otherwise medicines would be ineffective.

三 学术价值

如上所述，“戾气”学说的内容是相当全面的，它对传染病的主要特点基本上都论述到了，特别是在我国明朝没有显微镜观察到细菌、病毒等致病微生物的时代背景下，吴有性能够科学地预见其存在，并对温病的病因、传染途径等进行了有深刻见地的探索，为创立温病学说所做的贡献，的确是十分宝贵的。他是明末具有创新精神的著名医家，其所具备的创新思想和精神更应当赞扬，值得后人发扬光大。吴有性在温病学上所提出的卓见和诊治经验，丰富了温病学说的内容，为后来温病学说的发展和系统化奠定了基础。清朝温病学家在不同程度上受到了吴有性有关温病论述的启发和影响。总之，吴有性以他的医学实践和聪明才智在传染病学发展史上写下了宝贵的篇章，对传染疾病所进行的系统观察和研究，对其后温病学说的迅速发展产生了重大影响。

3 Academic value

In conclusion, the theory of "epidemic pathogen" is comprehensive in its content, which basically discusses the main characteristics of infectious diseases. It is indeed precious that Wu Youxing has made contributions to the establishment of the theory of warm diseases since he foresees the existence of pathogenic microorganism scientifically, particularly in the age that no microscope exists in the Ming Dynasty to observe bacteria and virus. He also explores the etiology and transmission routes of pestilence with profound insight. Being a prominent physician with innovative thinking, his creative idea and spirit should be given more compliment and carried forward by later generations. Excellent opinions and treating experience Wu Youxing proposes enrich the theory of warm diseases, laying a foundation for the development and systematization of warm diseases. Experts in this aspect in the Qing Dynasty have been inspired and influenced by his discussion on the warm diseases to different extent. In a word, Wu Youxing writes down precious articles in the history of infectious diseases with his medical practice and intelligence. His systematic observation and research on infectious diseases has produced a significant impact on the rapid development of the theory of warm diseases.

37 医林改错(Yilin Gaicuo)

Correction on Errors in Medical Works

一 书籍简介

《医林改错》是我国中医解剖学上具有重大革新意义的著作。作者王清任(公元1768年—1831年)二十岁左右开始学习医学,并逐渐成为当时的名医。他在长期行医的实践中,认识到要掌握好医学,首先要对人体脏器组织和功能有正确的了解,于是开始对解剖学加以研究。在研究中他发现前人的医著中对人体脏器的描述存在许多矛盾和错误,深感掌握正确的人体解剖知识对医家的极端重要性,于是他从30岁起经常到坟地、刑场观察尸体,面对被野狗撕咬残存的"破腹露脏"的病儿弃尸,"初未尝不掩鼻,后因念及古人所以错论脏腑,皆由未尝亲见,遂不避污秽"。通过长期观察,王清任绘制了人体内脏图形并以文字叙述脏器的生理结构,加上自己多年的临床经验,于1830年写成《医林改错》。他认为前世许多医书的讲法不正确,须改正,故书名便为《医林改错》。

1 A brief introduction to the book

Correction on Errors in Medical Works (*Yilin Gaicuo*) is a significant book with regenerated meaning on anatomy of TCM. The author Wang Qingren (1768—1831A. D.) began to learn medicine when he was about 20 years old and he gradually became a famous doctor at that time. During the long-time medicine practice, he recognized that only by forming proper understanding of visceral organs and functions of human body at the first step could we have a good command of medicine, and then he began to do research on anatomy. In his study, he found that many conflicts and errors were in the former medical books. Thus, he thought that it's extremely important for physicians to grasp correct knowledge of human anatomy. Then, he often came to cemetery and execution ground to observe dead body since he was 30 years old, facing sick children and deserted body remained after being eaten by wild dogs. "He observed it with his nose covered at the beginning. Later, he suspected that the ancient doctors made errors on zang-fu organs because they didn't see it by themselves. At the thought of which, he faced what he saw directly." Through observation for a long time, Wang Qingren drew pictures of internal organs of human body with description of their physical structures in words. Plus his clinical experience for many years, he compiled *Correction on Errors in Medical Works* in 1830. He thought that content in many former medical books were incorrect and had to be

王清任的《医林改错》是一部几百年来令医学界争论不休的书，对于他的评论历来不绝，褒贬不一，各有所重。然而历史的评价不应局限在结果的正确与否，而应重在他所表现出来的探索方向，因为这才能给我们以更深刻的多方面启迪。

corrected, so that was how the title of the book was nominated. It is a book with endless arguments for hundreds of years in the medical world. Various comments, with different emphasis, also have been made about the author Wang Qingren. The evaluation in history, however, should not confine to whether the result is correct or not. Instead, the direction of exploration he has reflected should be taken seriously. Only in this way can we get profound inspirations in many aspects.

二 主要内容

《医林改错》一书记载了许多之前医学书籍中所未能清晰描述的人体解剖内容，如书中正确记载了"人胸下膈膜一片，其薄如纸，最为坚实"的膈肌，这在中医学史上第一次描述了膈肌；同时他也指出了古人以往所记载的某些人体解剖方面的错误，如"肺有二十四孔"、"脾闻声则动"、"尿从粪中渗出"等，并加以纠正；他还明确肯定了脑主司思维记忆的功能，说："灵机记性，不在心在脑"。总之，王清任的这些积极探索对医学的发展是很有革新和进步意义的。

2 The main content

Correction on Errors in Medical Works records human anatomy that many former medical books have never described clearly. For example, "a diaphragm under the chest of human body is as thin as a piece of paper, but it's the strongest one", which has been the correct record and the first-ever description on diaphragm in the history of TCM. Meanwhile, he points out and corrects errors of record ancient people made on anatomy, such as "lungs have 24 orifices", "spleen transports and transforms food with sounds" and "urine effuses from excrement", etc. He also confirms that brain is in charge of thinking and memory, and asserts that "a keen memory lies in the brain rather than the heart". In a word, his active researches are of innovative and progressive significance for the development of medicine.

（1）补充大量解剖知识纠正以往解剖错误

本书约有1/3篇幅为解剖学内容，以作者的亲眼所见，辨认胸腹内脏器官，与古代解剖做比较，画出他自认为是正确的十三幅解剖图以改错。从一般的解剖形态结构

(1) Supplementing a large amount of anatomical knowledge and correcting anatomical errors in the former medical books

About one third of the book is about the anatomy. By seeing on his own, the author identifies internal viscera of chest and abdomen. Comparing with anatomy in the ancient time, he draws thirteen diagrams which he thinks right to correct errors. From the perspective of rough description on

及毗邻关系的大体描述方面看，王清任所改是十分准确的。他发现了颈总动脉、主动脉、腹腔静脉及全身血管之动静脉区分；描述了大网膜、小网膜、胰腺、胰管、胆总管、肝管、会厌及肝、胆、胃、肠、肾、膀胱等的形态和毗邻关系；描述了主动脉和静脉及其分支，气管两个分支插入两肺，胆总管及其开口、视神经等等丰富的解剖内容，同时他还创新性地提出了很多自己的见解，如否定天花病因的"胎毒论"；认为"抽风不是风"，是因"气虚而血瘀"造成等。

general anatomic structure and neighboring relationship, what Wang Qingren corrects is very accurate. He finds identification among common carotid artery, aortic arch and abdominal vein, as well as arteries and veins of vessels all over the body, describing shapes and adjoining relations of greater and lesser omentum, pancreas, pancreatic duct, choledochus, common hepatic duct, epiglottis, liver, gallbladder, stomach, intestines, kidney and bladder. Plenty knowledge of anatomy is also depicted such as aortic arch and vein, as well as their branches, two branches of windpipe inserting into two lungs, choledochus and its opening and optic nerves, etc. Meanwhile, he puts forward his own views. For example, He denies the cause of smallpox—"fetal toxicity", thinking that stroke is not wind, but caused by qi deficiency and blood stasis.

但由于王清任观察的尸体内脏多是残缺不全的，也由于受当时社会历史条件、文化传统和科学水平及其工作条件恶劣等多方面制约，他对不少器官的命名和功能解释以现代医学观点看是错误的。例如他将主要的动脉称为"气总管"、"气门"，并认为动脉内无血而有气，将主要静脉称为"荣总管"，认为血液及营养等靠它供应全身等等。对此也应当认识到作者所存在的局限性，因他不可能达到完全科学的观察和实验的程度，难免会存在某些认识方面的偏差。

From the view of modern medicine, however, his nomination and functional explanation for many organs are incorrect because the internal viscera of corpses that Wang Qingren has observed mostly are incomplete, and meanwhile his study is limited by social and historic conditions, cultural traditions and scientific level, as well as poor working conditions at the time. For instance, he calls the main artery "air general duct" or "air valve", and considering that there is no blood, but qi in the artery. He calls the main veins "*rong* general duct", thinking that distribution of blood and nutrition depends on it. Therefore, we should recognize the limitations of the author because the wholly scientific observation and experiment could not be conducted. It's hard to avoid some deviation in some aspects of cognition.

（2）在活血化瘀理论方面的重要贡献

(2) Important contributions in the theory of promoting blood circulation and removing blood stasis

由于作者在生理功能与

The author's new exploration and finding in the

解剖方面的新探索和发现，也使得他在活血化瘀理论及临床方面做出了相应的新贡献。他认为气与血皆为人体生命的源泉，但同时也是致病因素。不论外感内伤何种原因，对人体所造成的损伤，皆伤于气血而非脏腑。气有虚实，血有亏瘀。他认为瘀血是由于正气虚而推动无力造成的，故血瘀症皆属虚中夹实，故而他倡导"补气活血"和"逐瘀活血"两大法则，这就是他著名的"瘀血说"。书中约有一半以上的内容即为此而作。他所创立的通窍活血汤、血府逐瘀汤、膈下逐瘀汤、补阳还五汤、少腹逐瘀汤等活血逐瘀方剂，具有很好的活血通窍、活血祛瘀、活血通络功能，分别用来治疗50余种有关瘀血的病症以及半身不遂、痹症及难产等。这些方剂都是阐发前人之未发，且多可在临床上取得特殊的良效，至今被广泛应用于冠心病、中风后遗症等的临床治疗。该书对于中医学活血化瘀理论的建立具有重要的推动和影响作用。

physical function and anatomy also bring him new corresponding contributions in the theory of promoting blood circulation and removing blood stasis, as well as clinical practice. He thinks that qi and blood are sources of human lives, which are also the pathogenic factors at the same time. No matter what causes exogenous diseases or internal injuries, damages to human body lie in qi rather than zang-fu organs. Qi is deficient or excessive, so as blood. He thinks that blood stasis results from deficiency of healthy qi and inability to boost. Thus, the symptoms of blood stasis pertain to asthenia accompanied by sthenia. So he advocates two principles, including "invigorating qi and promoting blood circulation" and "removing stasis and invigorating blood circulation", which is his famous "theory of blood stasis" and occupies about over half of the whole content of the book. Prescriptions he creates for removing stasis and invigorating blood circulation are Orifice-Opening Blood-Activating Decoction, Blood House Stasis-Expelling Decoction, Infradiaphragmatic Stasis-Expelling Decoction, Yang-Tonifying Five-Returning Decoction, Lesser Abdomen Stasis-Expelling Decoction, etc. With great functions for activating blood, opening orifice, removing stasis and obstruction in channels, these recipes are respectively used for the treatment of over 50 symptoms about blood stasis, as well as hemiplegia, arthromyodynia and dystocia. These prescriptions are original ones that have never been put forward by former people, and most of which could have good effect in the clinical practice. They have been widely used to cure diseases like coronary heart diseases and stroke sequela in the clinical treatment. This book plays an important propelling and influential role for the establishment of the theory of promoting blood circulation and removing blood stasis.

三 学术价值

王清任是第一位对传统医学体系提出纠正的中国医

3 Academic value

Wang Qingren is the first Chinese doctor who strictly corrects the system of traditional medicine. After being

生，他的著作《医林改错》于1830年在北京刊行后，造成不小的震撼。该书自1830成书后到1950年间竟再版了40次，为古代任何一家之言的医学著作所不及，是影响一代医学思潮的重要书籍。

书中体现了可贵的不遵经、不崇古的创新精神，作者敢于向传统挑战，虽然由于时代的局限原因，书中也有某些错误认识，但是王清任在《医林改错》的自序里谦虚地声明："（书中）当尚有不实不尽之处，后人倘遇机会，亲见脏腑，精查增补，抑有幸矣"，表明王清任是抱着认真严谨的态度去开展脏腑探索工作的。他的这种勇敢追求科学真理的精神是应当给予充分评价的。

published in 1830 in Beijing, *Correction on Errors in Medical Works* brings a big shock to the mass. The book has been printed 40 times from 1830 to 1950, which are the most frequent among those written by all medical experts in the ancient times. It is an important book affecting medical thoughts of one generation.

The spirit of innovation, not sticking to rigid classics or following old thoughts has been exposed in the book. The author dares to challenge traditions though some misunderstandings do exist due to limited knowledge of the era. Wang Qingren states modestly in the preface: "There are still false points and uncompleted knowledge in the book. If the later people could have the chance to see zang-fu viscera by themselves, it would be fantastic to do a detailed exploration and supplemented work", which shows his rigorous attitude toward scientific research on the zang-fu viscera. His spirit to seek after scientific truth bravely should be given fully affirmation.

38 植物名实图考(Zhiwu Mingshi Tukao)

Illustrated Reference of Botanical Nomenclature

一 书籍简介

《植物名实图考》是一部关于植物研究的重要书籍。作者吴其濬(公元1789年—1874年)曾考取进士,先后任翰林院修撰、礼部尚书、侍郎、巡抚、总督等官职,到过山西、湖北、湖南、江西、浙江、福建、云南、贵州等地,有"宦迹半天下"之称。他本人对于植物学研究有浓厚兴趣,因此在各地任职与游历时,对当地的植物特别留意,观察、记录各种植物的生长和分布状况,大量采集植物标本,并经常向当地的民间医生和劳动群众请教,把采集来的植物标本绘制成图,通过多年积累,掌握了丰富的植物学知识。同时他又先后参考了多种古代药物学文献,汇集成《植物名实图考长编》22卷,后又在该书的基础上,进一步编著、修改和补充,终于写成《植物名实图考》38卷,是一部水平较高的植物学专著。

1 A brief introduction to the book

Illustrated Reference of Botanical Nomenclature (*Zhiwu Mingshi Tukao*) is an important book on plants research. Its author Wu Qijun (1789—1874 A. D.), a successful candidate in the highest imperial examination, had been successively charged as a compiler in imperial academy, director of the Board of Rites, vice minister, provincial governor and governor-general. Since he had visited Shanxi, Hubei, Hunan, Jiangxi, Zhejiang, Fujian, Yunnan, Guizhou and other places, Wu Qijun was praised as "an official whose trace of career covers over half of the country". With strong interest in plants research, he gave special attention to local plants when he took office and traveled in different places. Observing and recording their growth and distributed condition, taking notice of collecting numerous plant specimens, always asking for advice from local folk doctors and working people, he mapped those plant specimens. Thus, he had a good command of knowledge in botany through accumulation for many years. At the same time, he successively referred to various ancient literatures in pharmacology for compiling into 22 volumes of *Long Draft Edition of An Illustrated Book on Plants* (*Zhiwu Mingshi Tukao Changbian*). By further compilation, modification and complement, 38 volumes of *Long Draft Edition of An Illustrated Book on Plants* were completed eventually, which is a monograph on botany with higher level.

二 主要内容

《植物名实图考》图文并茂，书中所记录的植物均以作者野外实地观察所见为依据，参考相关药物学和植物学文献记述为辅。作者避免人云亦云，纠正了以往某些植物药的错误论述。例如在记述冬葵这一植物时指出冬葵“为百菜之主，……李时珍谓今人不复食，殊误……以一人所未食而曰今人皆不食，抑何过于自信耶?”作者强调医者应知药，认为医者不知药而用方是很盲目的，同时还批判古人所鼓吹的长服某些药物能成仙的谬论。

全书七万字左右，共 38 卷，记载植物 1 714 种，分谷、蔬、山草等十二类。每类列若干种，每种均详细记载名称、形态、产地、品种、性味、药用价值等，每种植物都附有较精细的插图，全书附图 1 800 多幅，参考文献 800 多种。作者对以往的药物学文献有匡谬，有补充，有发展，对于植物的药用价值以及同物异名或同名异物的考订尤为详细。作者本着严谨的科学态度，对于有些植物，虽经研究、比较，仍不能考订者，则一概不下结论。

2 The main content

Illustrated Reference of Botanical Nomenclature is characterized by the combination of pictures and texts. The plants recorded in the book were based on the site observation of the author when he was in the wild and with the reference to the related pharmacology and botany literature. The author avoided following the crowd and corrected wrong discussion on some former botanical drugs. For example, when he described the cluster mallow (dongkui), Wu Qijun pointed out that “it is the leader of all plants, . . . Li Shizhen said people today would never eat it, however, it is wrong. We cannot make a judgement that a plant is edible or not just because one person eat it or not. How could he be so sure?” The author emphasized that doctors should know medicines well. Otherwise, he thought, it’s indeed blind to make prescriptions without knowing drugs. He also criticized the fallacy that taking some medicines for a long time could turn people into immortals, which was advocated by ancient people.

With the total of about 70,000 words and 38 volumes, the book records 1,714 kinds of plants, which can be divided into 12 categories, such as grain, vegetables, mountain grass, etc. There are several kinds in each category. Name, shape, place of origin, variety, nature and flavor, and medical value of all plants are registered in detail. All plants are attached with exquisite illustrations, so there are more than 1,800 pictures and over 800 references in the book. The author corrects mistakes, adds and develops contents on the former medical literature, especially does the detailed correction on the medical value, synonym and homonym of plants. Since he holds rigorous attitude towards science, the author would not draw conclusions on some plants that still cannot be determined even with study and comparison.

三 学术价值

《植物名实图考》是我国19世纪一部科学价值很高的植物学著作。该书还保存了许多古代的植物、本草文献，又经作者分类整理编纂成书，为后人研究提供了丰富的资料，是一部很有参考研究价值的植物学资料汇编。书中对植物名称和实物进行了考证，使植物名与实一致，为植物学分类提供了宝贵的资料。书中所绘的植物形态图比较精细而近于真实；书中所记载的植物涉及我国十九个省，特别是云南、河南、贵州等省植物采集的比较多。所记载的植物在种类和地理分布上，都远远超过历代诸家本草著作，对我国近代植物分类学、近代中药学的发展都有很大影响。《植物名实图考》出版后，在学术上的影响比较大，至今仍是研究我国植物种属及其固有名称的重要参考资料，因此受到国内外学术界的重视。该书出版后，影响较大，曾流传到日本等一些国家，迄今不少国家的图书馆仍收藏有此书。

3 Academic value

Illustrated Reference of Botanical Nomenclature is a book on botany with high scientific value in the 19th century. The book preserves many ancient literatures on plants and herbs classified and compiled by the author. It is a compilation of materials on botany with great reference and research value, providing rich resources for later research. The names of plants and their real objects are verified to make the names in accordance with the real objects, offering precious reference materials to the classification of botany. The pictures of plants drawn in the book are exquisite and almost real. The recorded plants pertain to nineteen provinces in our country, among which, more plants are from Yunnan, Henan and Guizhou. As to the varieties and geographical distribution, the plants registered in this book far outweigh others recorded by physicians through the ages, which make great influence on the development of modern taxonomy and pharmacology and are still important references in studying varieties of plants and their inherent names. The publication of *Illustrated Reference of Botanical Nomenclature* makes greater impact on academy and is attached great importance both at home and abroad. Because of its great influence, the book has been introduced to some foreign countries like Japan and is collected in their libraries so far.

39 医学衷中参西录（Yixue Zhongzhong Canxi Lu）

Integrating Chinese and Western Medicine

一 书籍简介

20世纪初西方医学在中国的广泛传播和发展，促使一些思想开放的医家在吸收西方医学长处的基础上，努力探索沟通中西医学之可能，并著书立说，发表自己的观点和体会，形成了中西医汇通派。《医学衷中参西录》即是当时一部非常著名的中西汇通学术著作，是由当时的名医及中西医汇通派的著名代表张锡纯（公元1860年—1933年）所著。书中收录了大量的病例及方剂，以及张锡纯先生的评点文章。张锡纯幼时随父习文，数年后兼习医学，勤奋攻读十余年。由于他治病不拘一格，不仅能化裁古方，吸收各家精华，还能独出新意，融汇中西之长，使有些西医视为难治之症亦取得了疗效，在医学上声誉卓著。其一生从事临症和中西汇通工作，是我国医学史上一位捍卫与发扬中医学的杰出人物，当时的医界称其为"执全国医坛之牛耳者"。他将自己的心得体会撰

1 A brief introduction to the book

In the early 20th century, with the broad spread and development of western medicine in China, some open-minded doctors worked to explore the possibility of academic communication between Chinese and western medicine on the basis of absorbing the merits of Western medicine. They expressed their opinions by writing books and propounding theories, forming the integrative school of Chinese and Western medicine. *Integrating Chinese and Western Medicine* (*Yixue Zhongzhong Canxi Lu*), a famous academic work on integrative Chinese and Western at that time, was written by Zhang Xichun (1860—1933 A. D.) who was a representative of well-known doctors and integrative school of Chinese and Western medicine. A large number of medical cases of illness and prescriptions, as well as commented articles from Zhang Xichun, were included in the book. Zhang Xichun learned liberal arts from his father when he was a child. After years, he also studied medicine for decades. As he didn't stick to one pattern in treating patients, and he not only could revise ancient formula and absorb advantages from medical schools, but also could create new ideas and integrate the merits of Chinese and Western medicine, even cured diseases that physicians of Western medicine regarded as refractory cases. So that's why he got distinguished reputation in the medical field. Throughout his life, Zhang Xichun engaged in clinical differential diagnosis and integrative work between Chinese and Western medicine. He was one of the prominent people safeguarding and developing Chinese medicine in the history of medicine and was praised as "a pioneer of national medical forum" at that

写成医学论文，并汇集成《医学衷中参西录》一书，于1918年起问世，多次印行并广为流传，有很大声望和影响。

time. He compiled *Integrating Chinese and Western Medicine* in 1918 with medical essays written on the basis of his own experience. It was republished for many times and was widespread with great popularity and influence.

二 主要内容

《医学衷中参西录》共30卷，约80万字。书中结合中西医学理论和作者的医疗经验阐发医理，颇多独到见解。书中内容分为医方、药物、医论、医话和医案等部分，名曰"衷中参西"，意在初步尝试沟通中西医学理论。

2 The main content

Integrating Chinese and Western Medicine has 30 volumes in total, about 800,000 words. The book includes the principles of medical science by combining the theory of Chinese and Western medicine and author's medical experience, which is abundant in insightful views. Its content can be divided into prescriptions, medications, medical symposiums, medical professional essays and medical records. The title *Integrating Chinese and Western Medicine* aims to communicate the medical theory of Chinese and western preliminarily.

(1) 在思想理论方面倡导中西医理论相通

张锡纯三十岁以后才接触到西医学说，"颇喜其讲解新异，多出中医之外"，敢于抛弃崇古泥古、故步自封的观点，具有积极的创新精神。他指出："吾人生古人之后，贵发古人所未发，不可以古人之才智囿我，实贵以古人之才智启我，然后医学有进步也"。当时存在着中医基本理论方面如阴阳五行说与自然科学基本原理难通、藏象说与解剖生理难通、六气六淫说与微生物病因说难通、气化说与细胞说难通等问题。张锡纯在前人的基础上对这些问题做了大量的汇通探讨，经过十余年的探索研究，认为西医新异之理原多

(1) Advocating theory connectivity of the Chinese and Western medicine

Zhang Xichun got to know Western medicine in his thirties, "I am fond of its explanation because it is newfangled, which is different from TCM". He dared to abandon antiquated and conservative ideas and had innovative spirit. He pointed out that "Since I was born after the ancients, it's pretty meaningful to put forward something new. We should be inspired by what they have known, instead of being confined to their knowledge. Only in this way can the medicine be developed." At that time, there were many contradictions between the basic theories of TCM and Western medicine, such as yin-yang and five elements theory and basic principles of natural science, the visceral manifestation theory and anatomical physiology, six climatic factors and six exopathogens and etiological theory of microorganism, and qi transformation theory and cell theory. On the basis of the ancient research, Zhang Xichun made a large amount of discussion on these contradictions. He believed that the new and different points of view in Western medicine were actually included in the TCM after decades of exploration and research. For example, in his

在中医包括之中,如认为中医的“三焦”就是西医所谓的水道,《内经》中所描述的气血逆行于上而造成的厥证与西医的脑充血之论相符合,并指出中医的理论认识并不落后。

opinion, "*Sanjiao* (triple energizers)" in TCM referred to so-called water passage in the Western medicine. Syncope due to adverse flow of qi and blood described in *Internal Classic* was in accordance with encephalemia in Western medicine, which indicated that the theoretical knowledge in TCM did not fall behind.

(2) 践行医学临床 大胆并用中西药物

(2) Practicing clinical medicine and integrating Chinese and western medicine

对于中西医理论的汇通,他从临床实践出发,避免空谈观点,充分利用了长期临症实践的条件,尽一切可能通过切身体会去寻求知识。他认为学医的“第一层功夫在识药性……凡药皆自尝试”,自我尝试仍不得真知,则求助于他人之体会。因此张锡纯用药之专,用量之重,为常人所不及。如他充分发挥生石膏治热病的功效,改变了众多医家对生石膏的错误理解,张锡纯阐发此说不厌其繁,仅“石膏解”后所附医案即达38例,其中多系临床的危重症。他还创制了治疗霍乱的急救回生丹及防治兼用的卫生防疫宝丹。药味及制法系衷中参西的成果,经济简便而效果又在中西医之上。他所创制诸多方剂在治疗急症、防治霍乱等方面有所建树。书中张锡纯自拟方约200首,重要医论百余处,涉及中西医基础和临床大部分内容,几乎无一方、一药、一法、一论不结合临床治验进行说明。重要的方法所附医

For the integration of Chinese and Western medicine, Zhang Xichun made the best of his long-term clinical practice and did everything possible to seek for knowledge by himself, avoiding empty talk of opinions. He thought that "the first talent for people who learn medicine is to recognize the property of medicines… all need to be tasted by themselves." If we could not get the truth, then ask others for assistance. Therefore, he was better than others in the aspect of medication and dosage. For example, he made full leverage of gypsum that could cure fever, which changed mistaken understandings of many physicians. Zhang Xichun always expounded his opinion with great patience. There were as many as 38 medical cases attached to "explanation on gypsum", most of which were critical. He also created lifesaving pills that could cure cholera in emergency and anti-epidemic pills that could be used to treat and prevent diseases. The flavor and processing methods of these medicines were the result of integrating Chinese and Western medicine. They were not only economically convenient, but also more effective than either of Chinese and Western medicine. Many prescriptions he created made contributions to the treatment of emergent syndromes as well as cholera prevention and cure. In the book, there were about 200 recipes made by himself and over a hundred important TCM theories, covering basic knowledge in TCM and Western medicine, as well as most contents of clinical practice. Almost all prescriptions, medicines and theories were described according to his own clinical experience. Up

案多达数十例,重要的论点在几十年临症和著述中反复探讨,反复印证,不断深化。因此,张锡纯被尊称为"医学实验派大师"。

在临症上张氏大胆并用中西药物。他很推崇阿司匹林对于肺结核病的泻热作用,并主张将阿司匹林与玄参、沙参诸药合用以滋肺阴,"则结核易愈"。

to dozens of medical cases were supplemented to important methods; repetitive discussion, confirmation and deepening over important arguments were made in the following decades of clinical practice and medical writings. Therefore, Zhang Xichun was revered as "experimental master in medicine".

He was bold enough to integrate Chinese and western medicines in the clinical practice and praised highly the function of aspirin to purge the heat due to tuberculosis. He asserted that mixing aspirin with figwort root (xuanshen), the root of straight ladybell (shashen) and other medicines to nourish lung yin, then in this way could tuberculosis be cured easily.

三 学术价值

《医学衷中参西录》是张锡纯毕生心血的结晶,堪称理论联系实际的典范,全书逾百万言,学者多感百读不厌。书中内容多为生动详细的实践记录和总结,而绝少凿空臆说。书中作者自拟方剂大都被临床验证而有良效,故为不少医家推崇喜用。该书自刊出后也一版再版,流传甚广,影响甚大,当时各省立医药学校多以此为教材,时至今日,对于指导临床防病治病、科学研究,仍是不可多得的参考书。

《医学衷中参西录》体现了作者积极寻找西医与中医的共同之处的态度,认为"沟通中西原非难事",反映了作者从维护祖国医学遗产的立场出发,提出了"衷中参西"的主张,即以中医为本,来探索沟通中西之路。他从理论到临床,从诊断到治疗,均进行了汇通中西医的大胆探索,他的实践对当时及以后的医家都有很大的启发。

3 Academic value

Integrating Chinese and Western Medicine, the fruit of painstaking labor of Zhang Xichun's whole lifetime, can be said as the model integrating theories with practice. The scholars think the book, which is over millions of words, is worthy of repeated study and perusal. The book contains practical records and conclusions mostly with vivid and detailed contents, instead of empty talks. Most prescriptions made by the author are confirmed as good recipes in the clinical practice, thus they are preferred and used by many physicians. The book has been printed for many times, so it is of great influence with widespread publication. At that time, most provincial medical schools took it as the textbook. It is still a rare reference book for disease prevention and treatment and scientific research in the clinical practice till today.

The book reflects the author's positive attitude towards searching for common aspects between Chinese and Western medicine, holding that it is not difficult to integrate Chinese and Western medicine. It also embodies that the author explores the communicative approach on the basis of TCM from the standpoint of safeguarding the medical legacy. He takes bold exploration in integrating Chinese and Western medicine ranging from theory to clinical practice and from diagnosis to treatment. Therefore, physicians both at that time and in the later generations are all greatly inspired by his medical practice.

附录 1 常见中医典籍名中文、拼音、英文对照表（按拼音顺序）

书 名	拼 音	英 文
A		
敖氏伤寒金镜录	Aoshi Shanghan Jinjing Lu	Ao's Golden Mirror Records for Cold Damage
B		
八十一难	Bashiyi Nan	Eighty-One Difficult Issues
备急千金要方	Beiji Qianjin Yaofang	Essential Prescriptions Worth a Thousand Gold for Emergencies
本草纲目	Bencao Gangmu	Compendium of Materia Medica
本草经集注	Bencaojing Jizhu	Collective Commentaries on Classics of Materia Medica
本草拾遗	Bencao Shiyi	Supplement to Materia Medica
本草图经	Bencao Tujing	Illustrations on Materia Medica
痹论	Bi Lun	Discussion on Impediment
扁鹊神应针灸玉龙经	Bianque Shenying Zhenjiu Yulong Jing	Bian Que Responding to Jade Dragon Verses on Acu-moxibustion
扁鹊心书	Bianque Xinshu	Bian Que Heart Book
标幽赋	Biaoyou Fu	Ode to Reveal the Mysteries in Acupuncture
C		
巢氏病源	Chaoshi Bingyuan	Chao's Treatise on the Pathogenesis and Manifestations of Diseases
陈氏小儿按摩经	Chenshi Xiaoer Anmo Jing	Chen's Pediatric Massage
崔氏方	Cuishi Fang	Prescriptions of Cui Family
F		
妇人大全良方	Furen Daquan Liangfang	A Complete Collection of Effective Prescriptions for Women
H		
黄帝内经	Huangdi Neijing	Huangdi's Internal Classic
黄帝说	Huangdi Shuo	The Legends of Huangdi
黄帝阴阳	Huangdi Yinyang	Huangdi's Yin and Yang

续表

书名	拼音	英文
J		
金匮要略	Jingui Yaolüe	Synopsis of Prescriptions of the Golden Chamber
金针赋	Jinzhen Fu	Ode to Acupuncture Needle
经史证类备急本草	Jingshi Zhenglei Beiji Bencao	Classified Materia Medica from Historical Classics for Emergency
经效产宝	Jingxiao Chanbao	Valuable Experience in Obstetrics
景岳全书	Jingyue Quanshu	Jing Yue's Collected Works
救荒本草	Jiuhuang Bencao	Materia Medica for Famine Relief
K		
咳论	Ke Lun	Discussion on Cough
L		
雷公炮炙论	Leigong Paozhi Lun	Master Lei's Discourse on Medicinal Processing
理伤续断方	Lishang Xuduan Fang	Methods of Treating Traumas and Fractures
灵枢	Ling Shu	Miraculous Pivot
刘涓子鬼遗方	Liu Juanzi Gui Yi Fang	Liu Juanzi's Ghost-Bequeathed Prescriptions
M		
脉经	Mai Jing	Pulse Classic
名医别录	Mingyi Bielu	Miscellaneous Records of Famous Physicians
N		
难经	Nan Jing	Classic of Difficult Issues
纽伦堡药典	Niulunbao Yaodian	Nuremberg Pharmacopoeia
P		
普济方	Puji Fang	Formulary of Universal Relief
Q		
千金方	Qianjin Fang	Thousand Golden Prescriptions
千金翼方	Qianjin Yifang	Supplement to Essential Prescriptions Worth a Thousand Gold for Emergencies
S		
三十六难	Sanshiliu Nan	Thirty-Six Difficult Issues
三因极一病证方论	Sanyin Jiyi Bingzheng Fanglun	Treatise on the Three Categories of Pathogenic Factors and Prescriptions
伤寒论	Shanghan Lun	Treatise on Cold Damage

续表

书 名	拼 音	英 文
伤寒杂病论	Shanghan Zabing Lun	Treatise on Cold Damage and Miscellaneous Diseases
伤寒杂病论自序	Shanghan Zabing Lun Zixu	Preface of Treatise on Cold Damage and Miscellaneous Diseases
神农本草经	Shennong Bencao Jing	Shennong's Classic of Materia Medica
神应经	Shenying Jing	Classic on Acupuncture Points
食疗本草	Shiliao Bencao	Materia Medica for Dietotherapy
世医得效方	Shiyi Dexiao Fang	Effective Prescriptions Handed Down from Generations of Physicians
四库全书	Siku Quanshu	Complete Collection of the Four Treasures
四库全书总目	Siku Quanshu Zongmu	Catalog of the Complete Collection of the Four Treasures
素问	Su Wen	Plain Questions
T		
太平惠民和剂局方	Taiping Huimin Hejiju Fang	Formulary of the Bureau of Taiping People's Welfare Pharmacy
太平圣惠方	Taiping Shenghui Fang	Taiping Holy Prescriptions for Universal Relief
唐本草	Tang Ben Cao	Materia Medica of Tang Dynasty
通玄指要赋	Tongxuan Zhiyao Fu	Ode of the Essentials for Penetrating Mysteries
W		
外科正宗	Waike Zhengzong	Orthodox Manual of External Medicine
外台秘要	Waitai Miyao	Arcane Essentials from the Imperial Library
卫生针灸玄机秘要	Weisheng Zhenjiu Xuanji Miyao	Mystic Secrets of Health Acupuncture
瘟疫论	Wenyi Lun	Treatise on Pestilence
物种起源	Wuzhong Qiyuan	The Origin of Species
X		
仙授理伤续断秘方	Xianshou Lishang Xuduan Mifang	Secret Methods of Treating Traumas and Fractures
小儿药证直诀	Xiaoer Yaozheng Zhijue	Key to Medicines and Patterns of Children's Diseases
小品方	Xiaopin Fang	Classical Prescriptions
新修本草	Xinxiu Bencao	Newly Revised Materia Medica
洗冤集录	Xiyuan Jilu	Records of Washing Away of Wrong Cases
Y		
医方类聚	Yifang Leiju	Collection of Medical Prescriptions

续表

书　名	拼　音	英　文
医经小学	Yijing Xiaoxue	Beginner Books on Medical Classics
医林改错	Yilin Gaicuo	Correction on Errors in Medical Works
医心方	Yi Xin Fang	The Essence of Medicine and Therapeutic Methods
医学衷中参西录	Yixue Zhongzhong Canxi Lu	Integrating Chinese and Western Medicine
饮膳正要	Yinshan Zhengyao	Principles of Correct Diet
痈疽方	Yongju Fang	Prescriptions for Carbuncle
玉函方	Yu Han Fang	Medical Books
Z		
针灸大成	Zhenjiu Dacheng	Compendium of Acupuncture and Moxibustion
针灸甲乙经	Zhenjiu Jiayi Jing	A-B Classic of Acupuncture and Moxibustion
针灸聚英	Zhenjiu Juying	A Collection of Gems in Acupuncture and Moxibustion
证类本草	Zhenglei Bencao	Classified Materia Medica
植物名实图考	Zhiwu Mingshi Tukao	Illustrated Reference of Botanical Nomenclature
植物名实图考长编	Zhiwu Mingshi Tukao Changbian	Long Draft Edition of An Illustrated Book on Plants
肘后备急方	Zhouhou Beiji Fang	Handbook of Prescriptions for Emergency
肘后方	Zhouhou Fang	Handbook of Prescriptions
诸病源候论	Zhubing Yuanhou Lun	Treatise on the Pathogenesis and Manifestations of All Diseases

附录2 常用中药名中文、拼音、拉丁文、英文对照表（按拼音顺序）

汉语	拼音	拉丁文	英文
A			
艾叶	aiye	Artemisiae Argyi	argy wormwood leaf
阿魏	awei	Resina Ferulae	Chinese asafetida
安息香	anxixiang	Benzoinum	benzoin
B			
巴豆	badou	Fructus Crotonis	croton fruit
槟榔	binglang	Semen Arecae	areca nut
白术	baizhu	Rhizoma Atractylodis Macrocephalae	white atractylodes rhizome
薄荷	bohe	Herba Menthae	peppermint
C			
常山	changshan	Radix Dichroae	antifebrile dichroa root
草乌	caowu	Radix Aconiti Kusnezoffii	kusnezoff monkshood root
D			
大黄	dahuang	Radix et Rhizoma Rhei	rhubarb
大戟	daji	Euphorbia pekinensis	Peking euphorbia
当归	danggui	Radix Angelicae Sinensis	Chinese angelica
冬葵	dongkui	Melva crispa L.	cluster mallow
E			
阿胶	ejiao	Colla Corii Asini	donkey hide gelatin
F			
防风	fangfeng	Radix Saposhnikoviae	divaricate saposhnikovia root
防己	fangji	Radix Stephaniae Tetrandrae	fourstamen stephania root
茯苓	fuling	Poria cocos	Indian bread
G			
甘遂	gansui	Radix Euphorbiae Kansui	gansui root
干地黄	gandihuang	Radix Rehmanniae	dried rehmannia root

续表

汉 语	拼 音	拉丁文	英 文
葛根	gegen	Radix Puerariae	kudzuvine root
枸杞	gouqi	Fructus Lycii	barbary wolfberry fruit
H			
厚朴	houpo	Cortex Magnoliae Officinalis	officinal magnolia bark
胡椒	hujiao	Fructus Piperis Nigri	pepper fruit
黄连	huanglian	Rhizoma Coptidis	golden thread
黄芩	huangqin	Radix Scutellariae	baical skullcap root
J			
姜黄	jianghuang	Rhizoma Curcumae Longae	turmeric
L			
灵砂	lingsha	—— *	cinnabar artificial
藜芦	lilu	Veratrum nigrum L.	black false hellebore
刘寄奴	liujinu	Herba Artemisiae Anomalae	diverse wormwood herb
龙脑香	longnaoxiang	Borneolum Syntheticum	borneol
兰草	lancao	Eupatorium fortunei Turcz	bluegrass
M			
麻黄	mahuang	Herba Ephedrae	ephedra
曼陀罗	mantuoluo	Datura stramonium	jimsonweed
密陀僧	mituoseng	Lithargyrum	litharge
N			
牛膝	niuxi	Radix Achyranthis Bidentatae	twotoothed achyranthes root
Q			
青蒿	qinghao	Herba Artemisiae Annuae	sweet wormwood herb
茜草	qiancao	Radix Rubiae	madder
R			
人参	renshen	Radix Ginseng	ginseng
S			
三棱	sanleng	Rhizoma Sparganii	common buried rubber
桑牛	sangniu	Apripona gemari	mulberry longicorn
沙参	shashen	Adenophora stricta	the root of straight ladybell
山药	shanyao	Rhizoma Dioscoreae	common yam rhizome

* 表示拉丁文名称缺失。

续表

汉 语	拼 音	拉丁文	英 文
山茱萸	shanzhuyu	Fructus Corni	asiatic cornelian cherry fruit
商陆	shanglu	Radix Phytolaccae	pokeberry root
生地黄	shengdihuang	Radix Rehmanniae Recens	unprocessed rehmannia root
生姜	shengjiang	Rhizoma Zingiberis Recens	fresh ginger
熟地黄	shudihuang	Radix Rehmanniae Preparata	prepared rehmannia root
蜀漆	shuqi	——	sprout of antifebrile dichroa root
T			
菟丝子	tusizi	Semen Cuscutae	dodder seed
W			
五倍子	wubeizi	Galla Chinensis	gallnut
X			
雄黄	xionghuang	——	realgar
续断	xuduan	Radix Dipsaci	himalayan teasel root
玄参	xuanshen	Radix Scrophulariae	figwort root
血竭	xuejie	Sanguis Draconis	dragon's blood
Y			
茵陈	yinchen	Herba Artemisiae Scopariae	virgate wormwood herb
郁金	yujin	Radix Curcumae	turmeric root tuber
芫花	yuanhua	Flos Genkwa	lilac daphne flower bud
Z			
泽兰	zelan	Herba Lycopi	hirsute shiny bugleweed herb
泽泻	zexie	Rhizoma Alismatis	oriental waterplantain rhizome
知母	zhimu	Rhizoma Anemarrhenae	common anemarrhena rhizome
猪苓	zhuling	Polyporus Umbellatus	polyporus
竹茹	zhuru	Caulis Bambusae in Taenia	bamboo shavings
紫贝	zibei	——	Arabic cowry shell

附录3 常用方剂名中文、拼音、英文对照表（按拼音顺序）

方剂名	拼音	英文
A		
阿魏化坚膏	Awei Huajian Gao	Awei Hardness-Dissolving Paste
B		
补阳还五汤	Buyang Huanwu Tang	Yang-Tonifying Five-Returning Decoction
C		
葱白七味饮	Congbai Qiwei Yin	Scallion Decoction with Seven Ingredients
D		
导赤散	Daochi San	Redness-Removing Powder
独活寄生汤	Duhuo Jisheng Tang	Pubescent Angelica and Taxillus Decoction
F		
肥儿丸	Feier Wan	Chubby Child Pill
G		
膈下逐瘀汤	Gexia Zhuyu Tang	Infradiaphragmatic Stasis-Expelling Decoction
H		
和荣散坚丸	Herong Sanjian Wan	Relieving Swelling and Dissipating Hardness Pill
黑锡丹	Heixi Dan	Black Tin Pill
黄连解毒汤	Huanglian Jiedu Tang	Coptis Detoxification Decoction
活络丹	Huoluo Dan	Collaterals-Activating Pill
藿香正气散	Huoxiang Zhengqi San	Patchouli Qi-Righting Powder
J		
金匮肾气丸	Jingui Shenqi Wan	Golden Cabinet Kidney-qi Pill
K		
苦参汤	Kushen Tang	Radix Sophorae Flavescentis Soup
L		
六味地黄丸	Liuwei Dihuang Wan	Six-Ingredient Rehmannia Pill
M		
蜜煎导	Mijian Dao	Honey Suppository

续表

方剂名	拼音	英文
N		
牛黄清心丸	Niuhuang Qingxin Wan	Bovine Bezoar Heart-Cleaning Pill
S		
升麻葛根汤	Shengma Gegen Tang	Decoction of Rhizoma Cimicifugae and Radix Pueraia
少腹逐瘀汤	Shaofu Zhuyu Tang	Lesser Abdomen Stasis-Expelling Decoction
石膏汤	Shigao Tang	Gypsum Decoction
失笑散	Shixiao San	Powder for Dissipating Blood Stasis
四物汤	Siwu Tang	Four Ingredients Decoction
苏合香丸	Suhexiang Wan	Styrax Pill
T		
通窍活血汤	Tongqiao Huoxue Tang	Orifice-Opening Blood-Activating Decoction
W		
温脾汤	Wenpi Tang	Spleen-Warming Decoction
X		
犀角地黄汤	Xijiao Dihuang Tang	Rhinoceros Horn and Rehmannia Decoction
香连丸	Xianglian Wan	Aucklandia and Coptis Pill
逍遥散	Xiaoyao San	Peripatetic Powder
血府逐瘀汤	Xuefu Zhuyu Tang	Blood House Stasis-Expelling Decoction
Y		
异功散	Yigong San	Extraordinary Merit Powder
Z		
至宝丹	Zhibao Dan	Supreme Treasured Pill
紫雪丹	Zixue Dan	Purple Snowy Powder
左归丸	Zuogui Wan	Left-Restoring Pill